Doctor Assassin

A
Medical Science
Thriller

Mark R Belsky

ISBN 978-1-09839-488-2 (Print)
ISBN 978-1-09839-489-9 (eBook)

Published by BookBaby Publishing
Cover design by Rob Sturtz; Rob@digitalartist.com, www.SelfPubBookCovers.com
Back cover photo by Mark Karlsberg, Studio 11, Newton, Massachusetts

This novel is dedicated to the memory of a young cardiac surgeon who was killed by a patient's son. As a surgeon, I identified with his accessibility and vulnerability to the dissatisfied patient or family. Surgeons can save lives, but they are human too, and can only do what is humanly possible. They are given the gift to heal many, but not all.

To the loves of my life:
My wife Nancy, our children Scott, Julie, and Gila,
and our grandchildren.

CHAPTER 1

Poling into the short waiting line at Exhibition lift, Max spotted his prey over his shoulder, thirty meters behind. The early morning sun was bright, with no clouds to shield the rays, casting sharp shadows on the skiers. Aspen in the spring hosted the world's rich and famous and those who liked to ski near the glamorous people. Serious skiers also flocked to the challenges of March's deep moguls on the ungroomed runs.

The Saudi native's ski skills were impressive, as Max had expected. Although the target's homeland was a dry, flat desert over four thousand kilometers from the nearest European ski resorts, his skis sliced through the snow like a knife through whipped cream. Over the last three days, others stopped and admired his effortless, subtle movements; it was as if he had grown up on the mountains.

Max had to admit that it had been fun tailing his target over the most spectacular ski terrain in the United States. Nothing beats spring skiing with perfect weather in the Rockies. Although he'd rather be skiing with Lilah, if he had to work, this was a pretty good gig. The Saudi started each day leading his bodyguards down an intermediate slope, progressively advancing to steeper runs. The two guards fell behind, depending on wedge turns to keep from falling. They were obviously not in their element. The bulges on the left side of their ski jackets told Max that they were armed. The white jumpsuit effortlessly raced down the slopes carving perfect parallel turns in a tuck position.

The skier in white poled over from the Exhibition chair lift to the high-speed Loge Peak lift. He was heading for another hike up the Highland's bowl, a repeat of yesterday's assault on the mountain's steepest trail. Max followed from in front.

The watch on Max's wrist tracked the skier around the mountain. A tiny, translucent GPS transponder placed three days earlier on the back edge of the Saudi's skis allowed Max to see a red blinking dot on the Apple watch's map. Peering back at the target from ten chairs in front, Max exited the last station and poled further up the trail. With skis over his shoulder, he hiked for fifteen minutes up to the edge of the summit at Peak Gate, 12,350 feet above sea level. His eyes widened at the immense expanse of mountains.

There were no other skiers on the top as the group ahead of him had sailed down the slopes. Few dared to test the steep slopes in the early morning before the March sun had had time to soften the snow. This extreme environment invited Max to validate his training. He stood, deeply breathing in the cold air. Now he just had to wait for the target to reach the ridge.

For the moment, Max's thoughts drifted to his childhood. He had no shortage of internal voices to please—including his own. Necessity had made his father a militant defender of the State of Israel. He thought of his father, but also of his mother, a nurse practitioner who had spent her life delivering care to needy Palestinians. Rationalizing that this would be his last assignment, he sought to appease his reluctance to continue as a professional killer.

Peering down the mountain, Max saw the guards had dismounted at Exhibition lift and crossed over to Prospector for an easier way down. Alone, their boss skied over to the Loge Peak lift. Max anticipated a repeat of yesterday. The target climbed as he had before, trekking to the summit's edge for the forty-five-degree pitch slope, the steepest trail in the American West. With an eye across the ridge on the target, Max's competitive juices surged through his veins as he jumped over the edge. Sensing the Saudi would follow, Max sped down the steep mogul-strewn ski trail, Be One, baiting the target down the severe incline.

The Saudi ski racer strained to catch his breath. His legs moved as he commanded, but his heart pounded overworking to keep his form. His muscles screamed for more of the thin air.

No longer a conditioned collegiate downhill racer, the skier in white could not keep up and stopped to rest, as predicted, giving Max time to position himself. Camouflaged behind dense trees, he watched as the target had to turn left to avoid going over a snowless, rocky ledge. Max had an open shot. He reached inside his parka for the custom gun holstered against his chest.

As the target descended, not slowing to make the sharp left turn around the copse of trees, Max witnessed his startled grimace. Pointing the weapon, Max yelled, in Arabic, "Hey asshole, eat this," and squeezed the trigger.

A soft whoosh filled the air. There was no loud gunshot. The skier's damaged mouth stretched open as he screamed, and his eyes went wild transforming from outrage to panic in seconds. Thousands of tiny frozen projectiles of ice smashed into him, crushing the front of his neck and face, and dislodging the goggles with the force of a shotgun blast. Impact from the icy pellets made him gasp for air, and the uncontrolled momentum pushed him into a thick tree, knocking the unstrapped helmet off and flattening his face. His visage contorted in pain, but no noise could be heard from his wasted screams. Millions of frozen, one-millimeter spheres had destroyed his trachea and vocal cords. Crumpled on blood-stained snow at the base of the tree, the Saudi's remaining facial features bore a minimal resemblance to the image on Max's phone. The dying skier tried to lift his head, but the more he gasped for air, the more blood he inhaled, choking until he collapsed with his head twisted to the side.

Looking at his watch, Max waited four minutes to assure that the heart had stopped which he confirmed feeling no pulse in the dead man's wrist. He replaced the gun in the holster under his parka. The ski pass with no name hanging from the victim's neck made the assassin smile.

The kill had worked perfectly, with bruising and tiny holes in the neck with no residual buckshot. They would find him dead, and no one would know who he was until the police found his fingerprints in their databases. The Prime Minister had ordered the directed assassination, and the CIA, Interpol, MI5, and the Mossad could remove the name from their lists of most wanted criminals. Best of all, once the ice pellets melted, it would look like an accident.

Hidden in the shade of the trees, Max compressed a concealed button inside his sleeve. In seconds, his black helmet metamorphosed into a white one with two blue bands; his orange parka became sky blue, and his black pants changed to white to match his white skis. White parallel stripes appeared on his ski boots.

Max pushed off and continued down the mountain. In a few minutes, he passed the guards facing up the slope with lit cigarettes in their mouths, oblivious to what had happened above. Max said a mental thank you to RAMOW, who had built his ice pellet gun and chameleon ski suit. On his way down, he felt the exhilaration of a mission completed, and his focus shifted to getting out. He slowed as he neared the parking lot at the base of Aspen Highlands and saw his ride waiting.

Dani, the driver, had retrieved Max's bags from the hotel in Aspen and made the short trip over to the Highlands to pick him up. He waited at the bottom of the ski run in a midnight blue Lexus SUV. Dani was a *sayan*, a loyal member of the Israeli diaspora. Max valued his discretion. He opened the rear hatch and loaded the ski equipment while Max got into the back seat. As Dani drove out of the parking lot, Max furtively placed his gun in the locked carrying case and his ski outfit in another locked suitcase. He changed into casual clothes for the four-hour ride to the Denver airport. Max would have preferred headquarters' Gulfstream to aide his escape, but then he would have had to explain things to his friends in the CIA. The drive gave him time to think.

CHAPTER 2

SUNDAY, MARCH 5, 2017
ASPEN, COLORADO

The minimally-used trail delayed the discovery of the dead terrorist for thirty minutes. A 911 call notified Ethan, the senior patroller, that a skier was down on Be One. When the call came in, he had been coordinating the transport of a woman with a broken leg, who had fallen on Red Onion. The slain skier's location on the Highland Bowl slopes was on the opposite side of the ski resort. Ethan rushed to the Exhibition lift, connected to the Loge Peak lift, and a snowcat took him up to the Highland Bowl Ridge. On his way, he notified other patrollers to converge at the site for a likely resuscitation.

The transport was too small to ferry an injured skier down the mountain, so it had to make a return trip to gather the other patrollers and tow the sled. When Ethan arrived, he encountered a small group standing among trees around the fallen skier.

One bystander commented, "Look at all the blood covering that poor guy. He must have hit the tree really hard." Another onlooker turned away, bent over, and vomited at the sight.

One man shouted, "Where the hell is the ski patrol when you need them most?"

At that moment, Ethan worked his way through the crowd. He noticed the group seemed transfixed in horror and kept their distance. But he thought to himself, *Placing their ski jackets on the man in the snow would have kept him warm, if he were still alive.* Ethan made his way to the skier. In another minute, two more patrollers arrived to help.

The sight that greeted Ethan was not a pretty one. Despite that, he had to photograph the skier who lay crumpled on his back at the base of the tree, with his legs and skis unnaturally splayed. Grasping the man's wrist, he felt no pulse. The man wasn't breathing. No helmet or goggles remained on the crushed, bloody face. Black and blue bruises covered the victim's neck.

Meanwhile, Ethan's team of patrollers began the assigned tasks, cutting the parka open to expose a broad, muscular chest for EKG leads and started to attempt resuscitation. One patroller inserted an airway and connected a ventilation bag to force air into the lungs as another patroller began chest compressions. Ethan had seen skiers die from injuries on the slopes, but he had never found one dead upon his arrival. Despite this, he reminded his team that protocol required them to do everything they could. The chest compressions generated a pulse, but not when the team stopped pressing on the chest. An ampule of epinephrine injected into the heart didn't help. Ethan figured the head injury must have killed the man before anyone arrived.

The voice of the doctor in the medical clinic from the base of the mountain came over the radio, sounding tinny and sympathetic: "Despite the epinephrine, the EKG on our remote monitor confirms a flat line," it said. "Sorry, guys."

Ethan told his team what they already knew: "He's dead." Continuing the chest compressions nonetheless, the patrollers stared in silence for a moment, looking down at the body as the spectators slowly drifted away. He went on, "This is—*was*—a young, athletic guy; it's unlikely he died of a heart attack. The head injury and neck trauma must have killed him, compounded by asphyxiation." Ethan assigned positions on the sled, and they transported the man in the blood-stained white parka down the mountain, continuing the useless chest compressions.

By the time Ethan had found the victim, the assassin was already on the highway heading to the airport. As usual after a mission, Max was reviewing all elements of the kill. Everything had gone perfectly, Max's technique honed by eighteen years of experience as a *kidon*, a Mossad assassin. Never once had he felt any kind of ambivalence after a mission—until today. Why, he wondered as Dani sped towards the airport, had today's kill felt different?

CHAPTER 3

sam and Jibran, the dead skier's bodyguards, stood looking at each other at the confluence of several trails, called Prospector's Gulch. Nine months earlier, it had thrilled them to become Asif's bodyguards; they hadn't known that skiing in Colorado's mountains would be part of the deal. Despite having waited for him for almost an hour, smoking too many cigarettes, they were too scared of their employer to consider leaving.

"Where the fuck is he? He always does this…" Isam said in Arabic, stopping mid-sentence as a patrol sled sped by them, racing to the bottom. Suddenly, he recognized his boss's outfit. "Holy shit, look there!" he shouted, pointing his finger at a skier in a white jumpsuit lying on the medical evacuation sled. As the sled careened past, the patrollers were working on the man. Blankets covered most of the victim, but his boots and white snow pants were exposed.

Abandoning their cigarettes, the bodyguards followed well behind the sled. Neither of them said anything as they made their way down the mountain. They stopped at the bottom, where bystanders had gathered outside the clinic. Isam, who spoke more English than his counterpart, learned from one nosy man that the skier on the sled had lost control on a steep trail, hit a tree, and suffered severe injuries to his head and face. The guards lingered long enough to confirm the shocking news that their boss was dead.

"We are so screwed," Isam said to Jibran in Arabic.

"He brought it on himself," said Jibran grimly. "How could we have prevented what he did to himself?"

"Try telling that to his brother," responded Isam as he anxiously lit another cigarette.

"What are we going to do?" asked Jibran. Then he continued. "I hated the bastard, but I didn't want him to die on my watch."

"One thing for sure," Isam said, "we can't tell anyone about the booze and the drugs. I'm amazed he could ski at all after the cocaine this morning," he added, shaking his head. He then sighed, reached for his mobile phone, and made a call.

CHAPTER 4

Amir Khan sat in his home office reviewing the previous month's economic reports for the Kingdom. As Saudi Arabia's Minister for Economics, he had to sign off on the monthly reports before the King and the Prince saw them. When his iPhone rang, he didn't recognize the number but recognized the voice immediately.

"*As-salamu-alaykum*, sir, this is Isam." It was 9:00 p.m. in Riyadh but only 11:00 a.m. Mountain Standard Time in Colorado.

"*Wa alaykum as-salam,*" responded Amir.

Isam continued, "I am very sorry to inform you that, one hour ago, your brother died from a ski accident on the mountain."

Amir remained silent as he felt a sharp stab of pain deep in his gut. His head spun, and he felt lightheaded. He squeezed his eyes closed, but no tears came as crying didn't suit him. Not wanting to lose control in front of a subordinate, he took a quick deep breath and responded, "Isam, tell me what happened."

"Sir, he was found at the base of a large tree. Apparently, he skied right into it."

"Weren't you and Jibran with him at the time of the accident?"

After about five seconds of quiet, he repeated, increasingly angry, "Isam, did you hear my question?"

Isam stammered, "Sir… um, your brother had instructed us to wait halfway down the mountain. He wanted to ski alone down the very difficult trail. When your brother hit the tree, neither of us was with him. Except for skiing the steepest slopes, we were with him 24/7," he quickly added.

Amir felt like his brain was about to explode, but he kept his voice steady. "The two of you will bring my brother's body home. I'll make the arrangements for an airplane. Where are they keeping him now?"

"The ski patrol took your brother, praise Allah, to the medical clinic at the bottom of the mountain where he is now. I will find out if they keep him there."

"Good," Amir responded and then ended the call. He took several deep, shaky breaths, clenching and unclenching his fists.

Amir was dumbfounded. After all his brother had lived through, it was outrageous that he would die in a ski accident. Asif was an expert skier, for goodness' sake! Immediately, Amir feared that the truth would get out. What would their followers think if they learned that the fearless and much-feared Asif Ibn Khan had died while skiing in America? Amir could only share this information with Shazia, his twin sister. Outside the family and a few others, no one could find out what had happened. The world would learn that Asif ibn Khan had perished a martyr in the struggle for Islamic world dominance, no matter what. Amir gritted his teeth. He called to arrange his brother's return home and then reached out to his sister.

Amir looked around his office as his mind wandered. Looking at his watch, he stepped into a prayer room to perform Isha, the evening prayer, the fifth of his daily prayer rituals, as performed by the prophet Mohamed peace be upon him. Rinsing his hands, mouth, nose, arms to elbow, face, and then his feet, his ablutions were completed for prayer. Standing on his prayer rug cleansed, he placed his right hand over his left, covering his chest. Then, sequentially, as he had done since childhood, he repeated the

Qur'anic verses and prayers to Allah for each position, reaching prostration on the rug. His brother's feats were on his mind as he prayed.

Emotions arose in Amir as he tried to understand all that had changed in a matter of moments. He and Asif had spent many hours together planning missions and negotiating terms to assure their success in this room. Since their childhood, the larger and physically stronger Asif had bullied Amir. But in adulthood, Asif had been the willing provocateur of whatever violent acts Amir had dreamed up. Asif's aggressive nature propelled him to be the face of their organization. Hasan, their father, and the other four tribal leaders of the Salafi Mujahideen Cabinet had been more than happy to make Asif the nominal leader. Asif thrived on the affirmation he received from the movement's following. He recruited and trained many attackers to explode vests, leave bombs, or perform silent knife assaults. The loyal Sunni Muslims that the Salafi Mujahideen supported spanned much of the globe.

As he prayed, Amir thought back to a line of the Qur'an that he had quoted often to his brother: "Fight in the way of Allah against those who fight against you." He had always omitted the rest of the line: "But begin not hostilities. Lo! Allah loveth not aggressors."

As the sons of Hasan Khan, Asif and Amir had an ancestral relationship to the religious leader al-Wahhab, who had co-founded Saudi Arabia with Muhammad Ibn Saud 250 years earlier. In the last fifty years, the royal family had extended a privileged existence to the Khans, giving them a twenty-acre parcel of the desert landscape to build a residence in the prime Hitteen neighborhood of northeast Riyadh.

The King's generosity to Amir and his family was part of a longstanding unwritten understanding with the Khans. The Royal family would publicly deny all involvement with the family's organization while providing covert support for their activities. As so many of his fellow Muslims had long dreamed, Amir believed the caliphate was within reach. It saddened him that their father, with advanced dementia, could no longer appreciate all that his sons had accomplished.

Before his senescence, Hasan had been an imposing man. His official title had been Minister of Economics, but his primary responsibility was to instigate a war of terror against the infidels in Israel and the west. His fiery preaching had nurtured a jihadist mentality towards the movement's enemies, stirring up energy among the faithful for an armed struggle.

Hasan had welcomed his sons into the cabinet of tribal leaders after both had returned home following their college graduations in America. Amir had always preferred working behind the scene as the planner, whereas Asif—the daredevil—had served as the terrorist leader of the Salafi Mujahideen Cabinet's loyal followers. As the recruiter, Asif had trained future jihadists on how to shoot an AK-47 and make bombs.

Meanwhile, Shazia, their beloved sister, had pursued her work as a scientist at the King Abdullah International Medical Research Center (KAIMRC). She was a physician-researcher who had recently become Director of Riyadh's Virology center. For the sake of appearances, she kept a distance from the family's political activities.

Unlike Shazia, whom Amir saw as both role model and confidant, Asif had never filled him with a sense of closeness. Amir had tried not to think too hard about the details of his brother's violent exploits, even as he masterminded the logistics behind them. Whatever unease Amir had felt about Asif's subversive activities, his brother's ruthless commitment to their cause had allowed Amir to keep the blood of jihad off his own hands. But now, with his brother gone, he had to think out the subsequent steps to lead the Tribal Cabinet on his own.

Amir shook his head. He was getting ahead of himself and decided not to tell his father yet. Amir rolled up his prayer rug, took out his phone, and called Shazia.

CHAPTER 5

The mortality on Be One was the third skier fatality this year at the combined Aspen-Snowmass Ski Area. Within two hours of Asif's arrival at the clinic, the police had reported the incident and transferred his body to the Valley Hospital morgue. Because the ski mountain was on state land, the death was within the jurisdiction of the state police. The Aspen Police had no name to write in their report. They found $360 in cash in the man's pocket but no wallet and no identification. The captain who reported the death noted that this was the first John Doe he had ever pulled off a ski mountain. He notified the state police hoping they would take the case and spend their resources on an investigation. With an unidentified victim, the State Police had forwarded the report to the nearest FBI office in Denver.

The vibrating phone interrupted FBI Special Agent Walid Manzur from enjoying a typically quiet Sunday afternoon movie with his wife and mother. Looking at the screen, Manzur sighed and said, "I just got a priority message and have to go to work. I'm sorry."

His mother, Saira, who had lived with them in their modest four-bedroom home since they had moved from Boston ten years earlier, groaned sympathetically. She knew Walid was covering this Sunday for a subordinate who usually would have received the notification. "Too bad you have to work on a Sunday," she said. "I'll tell you what you miss."

Walid smiled and gave his taciturn wife a quick kiss on the forehead. He said to his mother as he strode to the door, "You know how it is, Mom."

Directing the Denver station and the region had its perks. The Colorado location of the FBI occupied a 220,000-square-foot, glass-enclosed structure built in 2010 on the former Stapleton International Airport site, northeast of downtown. From the corner office, Agent Manzur relished the picturesque backdrop of the Rocky Mountains. This year's mid-March snow depths had reached twenty feet, accumulating as high on the peaks as he had ever remembered. It was a far cry from Roxbury, a Boston neighborhood, where he had grown up. Today, the clear, blue sky exposed the three snow-covered mountain ranges. Twenty-five years of service to the FBI had earned him this.

Agent Walid Manzur drove to work, deep in thought. He had read the message and was skeptical. *What kind of guy skis at an expensive ski resort with no credit cards or driver's license on his person, only cash? A person who has someone else toting his stuff for him,* he thought. *Or perhaps he had left his ID in his hotel room. Was he trying to hide something?*

Walid had learned long ago that he must assume nothing. Unless he verified the facts in a case, he remained unconvinced. Something about this mysterious man's death seemed odd to him. At most major resorts, only two or three deaths a year occurred due to out-of-control skiers—and he couldn't remember a prior victim carrying no identification. Walid stared at the three pristine mountain ranges to the west as he called Aspen's Chief of Police, who had sent a message to arrange a meeting. He learned that the State Police were taking over for the Aspen Police and would meet his plane. *I'll have to fly up to Aspen and check this out,* he thought without satisfaction.

CHAPTER 6

As Instructed, Dani drove Max to Denver International Airport and dropped him off with only a small carry-on. The remaining equipment in the car would be retrieved on Tuesday morning before Dani's Aspen hair salon opened. During the four-hour ride, the two men had talked little.

"Dani," Max broke the silence, "I appreciate your driving me to the airport."

"No problem," said Dani, wondering, *Why this American doctor got courtesy privileges from the State of Israel?* He didn't know that Max worked for the Mossad. The short, slight, swarthy, dark-haired Dani had been born in Israel, which made him a *sabra*. A few years ago, a *katza*, a go-between for the Israeli secret service, had approached Dani, who had found it difficult to thrive as a salon owner in Tel Aviv. Since he was single, with no family obligations, he had jumped at the opportunity to move to the U.S. on the Mossad's dime and set up shop in Aspen. Ever since then, Dani had been a *sayan*, supporting Israeli activities around the world. After three years, he was financially independent—but he still upheld his obligation to serve, making himself available when requested for matters of state.

"Tell me about your place," Max changed the subject. "I understand you have built a successful hair salon business."

Surprised that the passenger had information about him, Dani became suspicious. "Yes, the place has been great. I had to arrange coverage to leave work in the middle of a busy Sunday." He switched the topic. "I hope your stay in Aspen has been successful. Do you come often?"

But Max reverted to asking about the hairstylist's career. "I'm glad things have worked well for you here. Why do you think you have been more successful here than when you worked in Tel Aviv?"

Dani was thinking, *How does this guy know my life story?* And yet, something in Max's sincere interest won him over. "They love my accent," Dani said with a chuckle. "The women think I'm Italian." Max smiled. "Tourists book their appointments months in advance. Aspen is a four-season resort and a fun place to live. I'm busy all year except April when I travel home."

They exchanged more small talk, and then Dani commented, "Those are cool skis you put in the car. Are they new?"

"They are a new Rossignol model," said Max. "If you want to borrow them for a few runs, please do. All I ask is that you have all my stuff at your salon for pickup Tuesday morning."

"Of course," Dani said, excited to use them tomorrow, his day off. And then, in Hebrew, he added, "Anything else I can do for you, sir?" It was a test; Dani was pretty sure that this American would not understand what he said.

To his surprise, Max responded in Hebrew, "Nothing else, and you do not have to call me, 'sir.'"

Max's response shook the *sayan*. The guy spoke English without an accent and Hebrew like a *sabra*! Dani kept his mouth shut for the rest of the ride. In the rearview mirror, his eyes widened as he watched his dark-haired, swarthy muscular passenger smoothly change his clothes in the tiny backseat. It was one smooth move. Dani felt intimidated by this man, but he was not sure why.

After getting out of the car at the airport, Max walked around to the driver's window, bent down, stared straight into Dani's eyes, and instructed him in Hebrew, "Have all my equipment in the salon ready for pickup no later than 8:00 Tuesday morning. Be sure not to open any of the locked bags." Dani nodded. Max put on dark glasses and a baseball cap and entered the terminal with his one small bag.

It was rare for Max to feel agitated when ending a mission. The well-planned assassination wasn't the reason—right? Killing a killer was something he had done many times. Constant vigilance was his normal state. Every passenger, every TSA worker, everyone who walked or sat nearby, was recorded in his memory. No, he thought, that wasn't the source of the stress. Something else was out of balance.

Among the late afternoon travelers at Denver's International Airport, Max sat quietly in one of the stiff terminal chairs, looking out the large, glass windows at vistas of the snow-covered mountain ranges and planes moving around the tarmac. He thought about what had made this mission different. For years, he traveled out of America and performed assignments in Europe, South America, and the Middle East. Each time, Max looked forward to returning to his adoptive hometown of Boston for joy and solace. Before today, he had always saved lives in his work as a surgeon in America; he had never ended them. The distance from his secret life had a calming effect. And now, assassinating a man on American soil had breached that boundary. He couldn't just go home to escape from his deadly actions. He was already home.

Max knew his mother would not have approved. Since the age of eleven at his mother's side, she provided primary healthcare to hundreds of Palestinians and Bedouins throughout the West Bank and Gaza. He always felt safe because the local population had respected her. Sarah may have been the only non-Muslim who traveled across these borders without fear for her safety. Seemingly unaffected by the tensions in the region, she ignored politics and embraced every person in God's image. When thanked for her care, she would respond, "It is my privilege to help you." One day, he'd told himself as a schoolboy, he would be like her.

Back then, Max wondered how his mother expressed love for the same people, some who were Israel's sworn enemies. He felt an ache in the pit of his stomach, knowing he could never have shared the Mossad part of his life with her. But Max asked himself. *If she had survived the attack—if she had seen what our family had suffered—would she have understood the reasons for my path? He sensed, Probably not.*

CHAPTER 7

On his thirteenth birthday, tradition invites a young Jewish man to read from the Torah, the Hebrew Bible. It was a special honor, and one Max took seriously, having had studied with a Rabbi for a year. His entire family, including both sets of grandparents, were in Jerusalem to witness this momentous celebration of Max becoming a man.

The ceremony to mark Max Dent's passage into adulthood began joyously. It thrilled Sarah and Solomon to have had their son's service performed at the Wailing Wall in Jerusalem, the holiest place in the world for Jews. After the men approached the Wall to recite prayers, the Rabbi invited Max to find his assigned Torah portion in the handwritten scroll and recite the verses.

Tall for his age and with precocious muscular development, Max appeared older than thirteen. He smiled to make sure his anxiety didn't show. He was proud to have his entire family present the first time he read from the Torah, just as his older brother, Bruce, had done two years before. At the end of the brief service, the chanting of old Hasidic melodies carried them a block away to a large banquet hall, serving multiple families for such occasions. His was the fourth of the day. The concurrent Bar Mitzvah celebrants were enjoying traditional food and wine at long rectangular steel tables. Photos of eighteen years of celebrations covered the dull, green walls. Two long steel tables with white tablecloths, plates, steel silverware, and balloons awaited the Dents' arrival.

The other families had finished their meals, laughed, hugged, and danced around their tables, singing traditional Israeli songs. Merriment filled the room. The Dent family and friends found their places at the two reserved tables in the center of the vast hall. Once they were all standing around the table, Max led the blessings. He sipped the sweet red wine, and all his guests cheered and began singing a celebratory chant of *"Sim'n Tov and Mazel Tov,"* a traditional Hebrew song of cheer.

Then, two small and seemingly inconsequential events took place that would weigh on Max for years. First, Max's Aunt Gila, his father's sister, excused herself to go to the bathroom, and her husband Samuel held her chair for her as she stood to leave. The singing continued. Amid the revelry, Second, Max's cloth napkin fell on the floor beneath the steel table. He couldn't reach it from his chair, so he squatted under the table to retrieve it.

With his head and shoulders covered by the table, Max did not see two Arab women walk into the middle of the restaurant. Dressed head to foot in black chadors with only their eyes showing, they tossed their backpacks on top of the Dents' tables. *"Allahu Akbar!"* they cried before triggering the bombs in the packs and their suicide vests.

Ears bursting from the fatal explosion, Max felt his body crushed under the table. As his hearing cleared, distant trident screams seemed to come closer. It took minutes before a server's powerful arms lifted the collapsed, heavy table for Max to crawl out, only for him to witness a horrific scene. His shoulder hurt badly where the table had fallen on him. With his ears still ringing, he couldn't focus. The man's forearms supported Max as he stood trembling. Many tables away, he saw people in dust-covered, torn suits and dresses, their mouths moving in expressions of anguish and horror. Temporarily deafened, he couldn't hear the intensity of their cries.

He looked to the tables where his family had been celebrating just moments earlier. No one was moving. Body parts were scattered everywhere.

The bomb had exploded right in front of his Uncle Samuel, causing the upper half of his body to disappear. The blast had flattened their tables, killing everyone else. Two seats away, his mother and father had crumpled in a pile on the floor. Max walked over to see them. Shuddering, he leaned to kiss their bloodied faces. His brother Bruce, on the other side of the table from Samuel, was dead as well. Max saw in a daze that both of Bruce's arms were missing. Feeling the blood drain from his head and face, about to faint, he bent over and vomited. That image would haunt Max for the rest of his life as he realized that Bruce had probably reached for the two backpacks.

Suddenly, Max felt Aunt Gila swoop in and grasp him in her arms. She had come running from the bathroom when the bombs had exploded. She embraced Max to her chest hard, sobbing loudly, screaming, "I can't find Samuel, my Samuel…"

Max's tears did not flow until the funeral, three days later, when he and Aunt Gila had buried eight family members. The depth of sadness they felt contrasted with the bright summer morning. After shoveling dirt onto all eight graves, Max sat on the ground for a long time at the cemetery. As he sat, his grief turned to rage at the fanatical violence of the Jew-haters, at the senselessness of all that loss.

After the funeral, Max had moved in with Aunt Gila in Ra'anana, a small suburb north of Tel Aviv. They were now each other's only family. It took a long time for Max to process the fact that his mother, father, brother, maternal grandparents, paternal grandparents, and uncle had died at the hands of Arab fanatics. How could these be the same people whom his mother had treated with such respect and care?

Nightmares full of loud screaming often interrupted Max's sleep. His mind swelled with the faces of the killers he'd never seen. Upon awakening from these dreams, he told himself many times that his mother would have said that these were not the same people she had helped. "Most people are peaceful," she used to tell him. "Only a few are fanatics." She may have been right—but his nightmares never went away. Absurdly, he blamed himself. If he hadn't had his bar mitzvah that day, his loved ones would still be alive.

CHAPTER 8

Max's flight home landed early. The double Johnny Walker Black Label scotch relaxed him and aided his sleep on the less than four-hour flight. A cab dropped him at his high-rise condominium building in Boston's seaport district. His excitement at coming home to Lilah softened his exhaustion. He got off the elevator and opened the door. Already after midnight, the sounds of Leonard Cohen filling the space surprised him. Lilah walked out of the bedroom in a tight T-shirt and skimpy undies; her long dark brown hair gathered in an adorable ponytail. Just three inches shorter than Max's six feet, she had a chiseled body, slender and shapely.

"It's great to have you home," Lilah said warmly. She walked up and hugged him. Max melted in her arms. All at once, the thoughts that had filled his head cleared.

Lilah's tight squeeze overwhelmed him. Her warmth aroused his love. Max lifted Lilah into his powerful arms, effortlessly carried her into the bedroom, and placed her on their bed.

Lilah watched as he slowly undressed, her arousal increasing. Max gently got into bed beside her. Their eyes locked on each other. Looking into her eyes, Max said, "I love you." In seconds, her underwear disappeared.

Awakening at their usual 5:30 a.m., Lilah turned on her side to see Max staring at the ceiling. "You didn't sleep well last night," Lilah said as a fact.

"What makes you say that?"

With a furrowed brow, she asked, "Did your nightmares return?"

Sheepishly, Max admitted, "Yes."

"What was it this time?" she asked, putting a gentle hand on his shoulder.

Max sighed, "You know—the explosion, the body parts, everything was there. It was so vivid. I couldn't fall back to sleep. But they're gone now. I'm okay."

Knowing the significance of this as only a psychiatrist could, Lilah said, "Max, I am trying to remember when the dreams last occurred. Wasn't it after your last trip?"

Max knew that his missions prompted recurring painful dreams of the attack. Feigning ignorance, he asked, "Is that what you recall?"

She made a stern face at him, to which Max answered, "Yes, could have been." Changing the subject, he said, "I'm hungry. Let's have breakfast together before we leave for the hospital."

Frustrated by his reluctance to explore his nightmares, Lilah knew better than to force him to confront them now. She got out of bed, threw on a bathrobe, and went into the kitchen to make coffee and egg white omelets. Her first patient visit would start at 9:00 a.m.

CHAPTER 9

t was cold, dark, and late when the two bodyguards completed packing up and leaving the rented home where the three of them had stayed. Isam and Jibran complied with the precise orders screamed into the phone by their employer's younger brother.

At 2:15 a.m., Jibran pulled a black Cadillac Escalade around to the back of the Aspen Valley Hospital into a parking space with a sign that read "Reserved for Hearse." A locked double door faced the spot. During a visit earlier in the evening, Isam had found the closed Pathology department and the morgue.

Jibran remained in the vehicle while Isam entered the hospital through the Emergency Department. Encountering lax security, he snuck away to the basement stairwell. Isam easily picked the lock of the Pathology Department door and found the morgue. A pungent, sickening smell hit him first. A glistening, tiled wall embraced six small, numbered steel refrigerator doors, three above three, each thirty inches tall and thirty-six inches wide. A white index card sat below each number. Only two doors held cards with names. Door number four had the name John Doe listed, and after the name, the word "skier."

Isam grimaced and shook his head at how ridiculous the situation seemed: his boss, one of the most ferocious killers in the Islamic world—and a champion skier—dying this way. After opening the refrigerator door, he pulled the cold, tray-like drawer out. It rolled on noisily grinding wheels, exposing a sheet-covered body with remnants of the white jumpsuit. Isam lifted the top of the navy-blue sheet. He barely recognized the crushed face with dried blood stains and bruises on the cheeks and chin. He shuddered. Where there were no bloodstains, his former boss's skin was pale white. Isam immediately recovered the body, then walked over to the end of the room and pushed open the double door.

Standing just outside, Jibran stared and froze. The foul smell caused him instant nausea. He had killed people, sure, but he had never walked inside a room like this. Staggering, he felt his face sweat. He could not find his balance as the room spun.

"Come this way," Isam grabbed Jibran by the shoulder and shook him, which helped him focus. Isam pushed a gurney alongside the body. The sheet slipped off as they positioned Asif for transfer. They both had to endure their boss staring at them with dead eyes. The stiffened body's weight made lifting it to the gurney difficult. Even in death, their boss's flattened face sent a message: *Look how you fucked up.* They rolled the loaded gurney out of the back door and lifted the body into the back of the SUV. Only the security cameras witnessed the theft. Isam returned the empty stretcher and closed the doors tightly.

"You'd better drive," said a light-headed Jibran as he climbed into the passenger seat of the SUV. His world was still spinning. Putting his head down between his knees, he turned sideways towards Isam. "I'm worried. What are we going to say when we get home?"

"We have to have the same story," insisted Isam. "Every morning, Asif ordered us to leave him alone to ski the steeper mountains and not to interfere. Forget that we hate skiing and didn't want to come on this fucking trip. And don't say he nosed cocaine before each day's skiing—that stays between us."

"What do you know of the younger brother? I hope he isn't a reckless asshole like Asif," said Jibran.

"He's supposed to be smarter," responded Isam. "The other guards never said much about him. Asif was the crazy brother. Life should be better off with Amir as our boss."

Jibran wasn't so sure. The cold, moonless March night chilled the two men as they drove the sixty-nine miles to Eagle County Regional Airport.

The bodyguards and the Saudi male flight attendants placed the skier's body into a black plastic bag and the bag into a large container. As Amir had instructed, they used 200 pounds of ice bags to preserve the body for examination by a Saudi pathologist. The guards closed the top of the makeshift casket. The plane flew out of Eagle before daylight.

No one enjoyed the eighteen-hour flight back to Riyadh, nor the lengthy stop in Greenland to refuel and pick up more ice. Despite Isam's encouraging words the night before, neither he nor Jibran had any idea what to expect from their new boss. They were exhausted but couldn't sleep.

"Don't worry, we didn't have a choice," said Isam to Jibran. They went over their story. "I hope the brother will find a way for us to continue working for their family."

Jibran muttered to himself, "Praise Allah, let him be good to us."

CHAPTER 10

MONDAY, MARCH 6, 2017
ASPEN, COLORADO

Monday morning, after a quick plane ride to Aspen, Agent Manzur climbed down the stair ramp and immediately noticed the somber face of the Colorado State Police supervisor, Captain William Rhinehart. "Thank you for meeting my plane this morning, sir. I'm Wally Manzur with the FBI."

Rhinehart's eyes took in this stocky, about six feet tall, olive-skinned man, as they shook hands. "Bill Rhinehart. Nice to meet you." And then, without a pause, he added, "I have bad news. The body's disappeared."

Manzur had sensed the moment he stepped off the plane that this man was not happy. Now he knew why. He asked, "What happened?"

"Last night, the hospital's security camera recorded two men taking the body out of the hospital's morgue at about 2:20 this morning. They used a back door near the hearse parking spot and rolled the body on a gurney into a rented black Cadillac Escalade. We found the car abandoned at Eagle Airport, rented under a false name. A private Gulfstream landed and took off around that time, but somehow, someone erased the flight plan from the Airport's computer records!"

Manzur's face intensified, and his eyes grew wider with each additional detail. Trying to stay calm and professional, Rhinehart continued,

"We're confident the stolen body left on the Gulfstream. The tail number was registered to an oil drilling company owned by the King of Saudi Arabia."

"Saudi Arabia?!" Manzur digested this news. Slowly nodding his head up and down with his chin in his hand, he said, "The mystery grows." He asked, "Did the ski patrol who found him or the doctor in the clinic take any photos?"

"I don't know. For major accidents, the patrol photographs the injured skier on the ground. I arranged for us to meet at the medical clinic first, followed by a meeting at the accident site. We can talk to the patrol there," said Rhinehart.

They spoke first with the physician who had treated the victim in the medical clinic at the mountain base. They also interviewed several nurses and medical assistants, but nobody offered any additional information. The only comment the trauma surgeon made was, "This was the worst neck and facial trauma I have ever seen on the mountain!" Afterward, they took a ride up the mountain.

On the noisy, bumpy snowcat ride up to Be One, Captain Rhinehart leaned over to speak into the FBI agent's ear. "The doc said the skier had died from direct trauma to his face and neck. He was skiing too fast. Since the victim is a John Doe, would the FBI be willing to take the case off our hands?"

"Yes, of course. We have more resources to help identify the guy," said Walid, appreciating Rhinehart's honesty. "I'd also like to review the videotape of the two men who stole the body."

Rhinehart responded, "I'll get that for you."

They remained quiet until they arrived at the spot in the woods on the steep trail where three ski patrollers were waiting. Yellow flags staked out the site.

"Thank you for agreeing to meet with us," Captain Rhinehart said to the patrollers.

Manzur introduced himself and said, "Please tell us what happened. Start from the beginning. How were you notified to come to this spot?"

Ethan retold the story, adding at the end, "The victim never responded to the resuscitation. "The doc in the medical clinic radioed up to us on the mountain that the guy was flatlining." The other three patrollers had nothing to add.

Walid said, "Please show me the photos you took."

Ethan retrieved the small digital camera from his backpack. He flipped through the photos and then suddenly grimaced. "Here is the poor guy," said Ethan. "There are two or three from different angles. With the snow background, the white balance in my automatic camera darkens the face."

After studying the images in the camera, Manzur requested, "I'd like to borrow the SD card in your camera if that's all right. I will return the card to you with all the other images."

"Sure," said Ethan. "I assume the FBI is here because this victim had no identification?"

"Exactly." Manzur paused and stared at the images, his stomach turning as he imagined hitting the tree face-first. The FBI agent studied the terrain. Then Manzur asked Ethan to climb up the slope and position himself where the skier would have come from before hitting the tree. He asked Ethan to ski with some speed down around the bend and end up in the spot where they had found the victim.

Ethan obliged. He gathered speed and made the same left turn around the copse of trees. Walid asked, "If you were going too fast curving around the trees and lost control, what do you think you would have done?"

"Aimed up the slope to the left of the tree to slow down," pointing with his finger, "and gone into those bushes over there. I would have done anything to avoid hitting that tree," Ethan said.

"I agree," said Walid, who had taken out his cell phone and snapped a half-dozen more images. His mind was a pressure cooker of suspicions as he assessed the scene. There was plenty of space upslope of the tree, and the skier could have swerved to avoid it. Why hadn't he? Manzur thought to himself that the skier must have been unable to react in time. *Was he drugged? But he had made it this far down a treacherous run. Did something happen to him acutely? Like a heart attack, a burst aneurysm, or something else?* Manzur's thoughts raced.

"Thank you, everybody, for coming here," said Manzur. "I am returning to my office in Denver. If any of you have other thoughts or ideas we didn't cover, here is my card. Ethan, I'll send your SD card tomorrow."

During his flight back to Denver and drive to the office, Walid realized *he might have the murder of an unknown victim to solve.* His first thought was to send Ethan's photos to his superior, Thomas "Smitty" Smith, the Special Agent in Charge of the Washington, DC office. As the temporary SAC for the FBI's Middle Eastern Desk, Manzur hoped that Smitty might have some thoughts on how the jet from Saudi Arabia fit in.

Later that day, once he was back in his office, he made the call. "Hey, Smitty, this is Wally Manzur in Denver."

"Hi, Wally. How are things in Denver? I hope your family is well."

"Thank you, Smitty. I appreciate your thoughts. Work is my escape. My mother, Saira, lives with us. Fiona is still having a tough time; she misses our son. She needs Saira's support to get through each day."

He switched gears abruptly. "Anyway, look, the reason I called: I need some help to identify a deceased skier found by the ski patrol on the mountain yesterday. He had no ID. This morning, I flew up to the mountain. I learned two men stole the body and flew it on a Gulfstream with a Saudi Arabia registry. The videotapes from the hospital revealed two men taking the body out on a gurney into a black Escalade. Since it was at night, their faces appeared dark. I'll get some improved facial images of the two men from the tape and will send them to you as well. The trail ends at Eagle Airport, where they abandoned their rented SUV."

"Yes, I received the photo you sent me. Not a pretty sight. The lab will work on this for identity and follow up with you."

"Thanks, Smitty—and, just one more thing," said Walid. "I don't think this was an accident."

A note of interest entered Smitty's voice. "What did you find?"

Manzur reviewed with Smitty what he had learned on the mountain. He also acknowledged there was no body, no weapon, and no suspect.

"Wally," Smitty said grimly, "you don't have much."

"I know. I'm returning to the mountain tomorrow with a couple of analysts. We plan to try out the new facial recognition software to study the mountain's videotapes. I've got to figure this out."

"Good luck. If I learn anything about the victim, I'll contact you," said Smitty. Then he hung up, leaving Manzur alone with his thoughts.

CHAPTER 11

Back in Boston, Dr. Dent was about to start his fourth heart surgery case of the day, all part of an average day's work. The first three surgeries, each with a valve replacement and three coronary artery bypass grafts, ran on time and without difficulties. Max was relieved that the crew had kept its efficiency despite David's absence. For seven years, David Springs, R.N. had worked with Max to build the cardiac team of surgical nurses, pump technicians, and assistants, serving as their leader for all of Dr. Dent's cases. His nickname was the Checklist Master. Being detail-oriented suited him, as he reminded everyone to tick off each line item in the list on the wall before starting surgery and before any of the high-risk steps.

Springs hadn't shown up for work today, and he hadn't called out sick, either. He'd never done that before. They missed his presence but plowed through the cases without their senior surgical nurse present. They followed the checklist cursorily, not as conscientiously as David would have demanded.

Max enjoyed working with this year's cardiac fellow who was nearing the end of his three-month rotation. Having impressed Max, the young surgeon welcomed the privilege of starting the case and opening the chest. Eager to prove himself, the fellow rushed through the checklist, prepped, and draped the patient, and began the procedure by opening the woman's sternum and exposing the heart. He cross-clamped the aorta, stopping the natural flow of blood from the heart to all the organs in the body, including the brain. As he opened the cannula from the pump into the aorta, placing the patient on bypass, Max entered the room, gowned, and gloved.

Suddenly, the senior pump technician exclaimed, "No blood flow!" The fellow froze. The two technicians started yelling at each other to do something. Lack of blood flow couldn't continue for long because the patient wasn't receiving any oxygen to the brain.

Max looked at the heart pump, and without raising his voice, demanded, "How much heparin did you inject?"

The fellow's face reddened as he realized his mistake: he had forgotten to ask for an injection of the critical blood thinner. Sheepishly, he said, "I forgot." *If David had been there,* thought Max, *this never would have happened.*

Despite being in gown and gloves, Max lithely knelt on the floor in front of the pump and removed all the clotted tubing and plastic pump parts while requesting that the pump technicians retrieve a replacement set. Simultaneously, he instructed the anesthesiologist to inject 10,000 units of heparin intravenously and place the patient on 100% oxygen.

He ordered the fellow to remove the cross-clamp on the aorta and begin cardiac massage to circulate the heparinized blood through the patient. Max reassembled the cardiac bypass pump in less than ninety seconds. He told the technicians to load another 10,000 units of heparin into the pump, add two units of blood into a fresh batch of Del Nido's solution, which would mix with the patient's blood in the bypass machine. Max stood up once the pump was primed; the second scrub nurse assisted with a new gown and gloves. Standing at the OR table, on the other side of the patient, Dr. Dent had the fellow to cross-clamp the aorta again and place the beating heart on by-pass.

The anesthesiologist reported that the monitoring EEG on the patient's scalp documented no evidence of injury to the brain. At that, the entire team breathed a collective sigh of relief. The bypass had worked, and the patient hadn't suffered from the error. Max lifted his head to the cardiac surgery fellow who had been deathly quiet since this near-catastrophe.

"Okay, let's finish the operation we planned for Mrs. Collins today." The fellow expected his boss to take over, but Max said, "Carry on." He didn't want to humiliate the guy. Fortunately, the rest of the case went well, and the patient awakened with no complications. *Thank God*, thought Max.

He left the operating room, chatted with the fellow, called Mrs. Collins' family, and stopped at the main OR desk. He learned that David had not answered his cell phone, which was strange, not like David at all.

"Sheila, we should reach out to David's brother," Max told the nurse manager at the OR main desk. "He is the only family David has since he broke up with his partner last year. I think I remember David telling us he had planned a long weekend away in St. Thomas." Max tried to remember the details; at the time, the conversation had felt so innocuous. "I suspect he traveled with friends," Max said. "Can you text me the cell number for David's brother?"

Max stepped outside, into the hospital courtyard, and found the phone number he needed. David's brother picked up on the first ring.

"Hello, this is Dr. Max Dent. I am calling to see if you know where David is. He didn't show up for..."

Interrupting Max, David's brother spoke in a pained voice, struggling to form the words, "The St. Thomas police just hung up. They told me..." Max heard loud sobbing over the phone, and then the brother continued: "They found David dead in his bed yesterday, Sunday morning. They think he died in his sleep. The police officer gave me no details." Neither he nor Max said anything for a long moment. Then he went on. "I can't believe it. This whole thing sounds unbelievable." Max heard David's brother crying uncontrollably.

"I am so sorry," Max said, still letting the weight of the news sink in. His immediate thought was a practical one: they would need an autopsy to figure this out. But what he said was, "David was an exceptional nurse, an invaluable member of our team. And such a good person, too. I am truly sorry." Then Max said, "Did they say anything about when they were sending David's body home for a funeral?"

"No." Between tears, David's brother answered, "They told me I had to go to St. Thomas to identify David before that could happen. Silence followed before he added, "I can't do that. He is—was—the professional in our family. My wife and I are artists. This whole thing scares me; I'm no use in these situations…" Max heard the tears filling the man's throat again, "Flying to some island is out of the question. I can't." His voice broke, and loud sobs filled the phone's earpiece again. Max let the brother cry, thinking about what to do.

"What if I went to St. Thomas to identify David and brought him home?" asked Max.

There was a dramatic pause in the crying. "Um, sure." David's brother said, surprised. "You would go down there for me?"

"Yes, of course," Max said, half-surprised at himself. "I would go for you *and* David. He was a critical member of our surgical team. We got close over the years. Since he and Marshall broke up, he was not alone in his melancholy. He spoke with me and others on the team about his sadness." Max sighed. "We missed him today, and he will be hard to replace. The least I can do is help."

"Thank you, Dr. Dent. I can't thank you enough," said David's brother. Then he asked abruptly, "You don't think he committed suicide?"

"I very much doubt that. David was in pain from the breakup, but he still had his upbeat spirit. And I know he was excited about the trip. I'll find out what I can when I get to St. Thomas."

"The St. Thomas police are emailing me some paperwork. I'll forward the information to you, signed, so they will allow you to claim David's body. It's all so painful."

"I know," Max said. "Sudden losses just feel unreal at first." Then he promised, "I'll fly out tomorrow morning and call you from St. Thomas when I have things figured out."

In his Porsche, Max picked up Lilah at their waterfront apartment and drove to Brookline for an early dinner at Zaftigs. He related the story about David Springs to her but didn't share his heroics in the OR. He looked over at her as they got out of the car and felt a surge of love. Goosebumps formed down his spine staring at her large brown eyes and full-lipped smile.

Waiting for them at their usual table was Shalom. The older barrel-chested gray-haired man, speaking in Hebrew, greeted them in his gravelly voice, "I am so glad you agreed to eat with me this afternoon." Shalom hugged Lilah first, then bearhugged Max as he whispered into his ear.

"Uncle Shalom, what a pleasant surprise," Lilah said as she bit her lip and looked askance at Max.

"Just don't tell Miriam," Shalom smiled, pointing a finger as he instructed Lilah and Max, "that I am here enjoying their hot pastrami. She says it aggravates my diverticulitis! But what does she know, she's no doctor!"

Max replied, "Miriam is probably right."

Lilah got up, "I'm going to the lady's room while you two talk about what you need to discuss," said with a wry smile.

Shalom began, "How did she know…?"

"Your whispering in my ear was pretty obvious," said Max. "What's up?"

"Rosh insists you return to HQ. They need you to solve a problem. I don't know any details."

Max responded in a calm but clear voice. "I told Rosh that Aspen was my last mission. My life is here now."

"Didn't you get HQ's signal to come home?" Shalom asked incredulously.

"I got the signal on my phone, but I ignored it," Max said dismissively.

Staring into Max's face, Shalom insisted, "Max, something big is going down. You are the best at resolving these international threats. You should at least give Rosh the courtesy of a visit."

"I thought you said you knew no details," Max said, sitting up in his chair and moving his head closer. Shalom had been Max's father's best friend. Max loved him like family. His bar mitsvah occurred while Shalom was on a year's-long assignment in France. Over the years, he had shepherded Max's evolution into the Mossad and became his *katza*, his handler. Coincidentally when Max had moved to the U.S., Shalom's son, a dentist, had moved with his wife and children to the Boston area. Although always happy to see his *katza*, Max certainly did not welcome Shalom's news.

Lilah made her way back to the table and said, "Time out! I'm back. Does anyone want to eat? I'm starved. And where are the pickles?"

"Sorry about that," Max spoke first, "I forgot to order the pickles." Max raised a hand, and a waitress rushed over to their table.

Once the waitress had taken the order and left, Max looked into Lila's brilliant, dark brown eyes and said, "Some women, when pregnant, yearn for pickles. Could that be the case?" Max shot her a wide smile

"Not a chance," Lilah said with a mischievous grin. "I love pickles when I'm in a deli. That's it." The half barrel of pickles arrived. She took a bite out of a half-sour and chewed, still smiling. Holding the pickle in her hand and pointing it at Max, "Besides, before I had children, I'd have to be married. What makes you think I want to have yours?"

Ouch! Bullseye on that response! Max smiled at how she could startle him. Lilah swallowed her bite and changed the subject. Looking at Shalom, she said, "So, Shalom, did you hear that our hero," still pointing the pickle at Max, "is flying tomorrow to St. Thomas? His surgical team nurse died on vacation, and Max is jetting down to help the family bring back the body." Turning back to Max, "How can you drop everything and go?"

"The simple answer is, because I can and because it's the right thing to do for David and his family. Besides, had David been in the OR today, we would have avoided a near-catastrophe." Lilah looked concerned at this, but Max brushed it off. "Not to worry; it all ended up fine. But anyway," Max took a sip of his cream soda, "Now David is dead with no logical explanation."

The server brought a tray of food. Shalom grabbed half his sandwich and started devouring it. Russian dressing dripping down from both corners of his mouth as if it were his first meal in a month.

Wiping his face with a napkin but missing most of the dressing on his cheeks, Shalom spoke up, "Max, you have more important things to do. Send somebody else." Max did not appreciate Shalom's comment, and his face let the older man know.

"But David's sudden death makes no sense! I need to go there. I'll identify David and return with his body on the next flight." But he was already thinking about the situation in Tel Aviv. He looked down at his plate, less hungry than when he had ordered.

CHAPTER 12

Low-lying thick clouds dulled the morning light and drifted south over northern Germany, dropping light, steady snow. The frigid sea breeze made the drive to the Institute more treacherous, but Dr. Jaeger Brandt's mood as he hummed his favorite Haydn tune was more pleasant than the ominous weather.

The night before, he had returned from a brief trip to a tropical climate. The return had required sixteen hours of travel involving two airplanes and a long cab ride from Berlin. Arriving at his well-restored, pre-World War II apartment building in the village of Greifswald had been a relief. He had accomplished what he set out to do.

Dr. Brandt's typical morning drive to the Institute where he had worked for thirteen years took twenty-two minutes. His dark green BMW 7 Series sedan slowed and crossed the narrow causeway. Jaeger marveled at the German nation's foresight. In 1910, they had built the world's first institute to study viruses on the Isle of Riems along the northeastern coast of Germany, isolating the laboratories from the rest of the country. Since the 1970s, a 1,000-meter gated causeway passed over a dam and separated the rest of the country from the island and the top-secret scientific experiments conducted there. Peeking in his rearview mirror, Jaeger's prideful smile reflected the power he felt. Even his uncle Franz had never attained the recognition that would soon be his.

The Friedrich-Loeffler Institute, Germany's National Institute for Animal Health, employed 850 scientists, technicians, and administrators who conducted research to protect humans and animals from infections. The Institute housed several Biosafety Level 4 Laboratories to study the world's most dangerous infectious diseases. In case of an outbreak, the guards could close the bridge, cutting off the only road access between the island and mainland Germany. The Isle belonged to the city of Greifswald, but it felt like a secret world of its own.

Wearing a heavy leather overcoat over his tailored three-piece suit and starched white shirt, his dark blue tie tied in a perfect Windsor knot and matching his icy blue eyes, Jaeger marched through the front door of the building. Impeccable taste in conservative dress came naturally to him. A livelier pace replaced his usual, metronome-like cadence, precisely, step after step.

Jaeger stopped at the public relations receptionist's counter and deliberately said hello to Sylvia, the woman on duty. Greeting Sylvia was something he had never done before, but today he was generous. The upcoming meeting would be his time in the spotlight, his chance to show the successful results of his second clinical trial. Smiling to himself, he thought, *It will knock their socks off.*

It had taken Jaeger years to perfect his unique virology techniques, and now, at last, he was approaching the fulfillment of his childhood dream. The initial phase of the experiment, including the trial in Atlanta, had proceeded as planned. The plan for Phase Two had been simple to arrange. Of course, four travel days back and forth to the horrible location in the tropical islands made the trip barely tolerable. He hated the steamy weather and the people. But by doing the trials outside of Europe, Jaeger had identified easier targets and minimized collateral risk. He figured that if he had failed, then he'd hurt no one of significance. It had all gone so easily, he thought, smiling to himself.

Dr. Brandt's upbeat approach to Sylvia's public relations counter surprised her. He had never acknowledged her presence in the four years she'd worked the desk. She wondered if this change in Brandt's behavior meant something. She made a mental note to herself: *When I get home, I will send an incident report to my handler.* But all she had said to Jaeger was, "Good morning, Herr Doctor Brandt. Have a lovely day!"

CHAPTER 13

MONDAY, MARCH 6, 2017
RIYADH, SAUDI ARABIA

The following day, Amir, in his long flowing white thwab, covering him from neck to ankles, with his typical red and white checkered headscarf and open-toed leather sandals, left his home office accompanied by two guards and walked one hundred meters to his father's home. The short walk seemed longer as if the shoes he now wore were much larger and heavier than before. He now lived in a world without Asif's protection.

As he climbed the last few steps into his father's walled-off residence, he wondered, *Will I be able to demand respect, to lead?* There was no one left to show him how.

The guards waited out front while Amir ascended the stairs to his father's bedroom. Hasan's dementia had progressed to where he no longer went out. Straps across the chest and lap held him upright in a wheelchair. A woman spooned an orange-colored puree, the consistency of baby food, between his open lips. Orange drool dripped from the edges of his mouth. Watching this, Amir was glad he didn't have to visit more than once a week. This man may have been his father, but there wasn't much of him left. Another servant woman was tidying up the bedsheets. Amir stared at the two women. They stopped the tasks they were performing for Hasan and left the room, closing the door.

Amir addressed the man in the wheelchair.

"How are you feeling today, father?"

There was no response as the non-blinking dark and deep-set eyes stared straight ahead. His face sagged in constant sadness.

"Something terrible has happened," Amir said. The elder's face remained fixed. "I am sad to tell you, father, that Asif has died." Amir continued staring at the blank but vaguely sad face. Slowly, from one eye, a few tears made their way down his father's cheek.

Stepping closer to Hasan, as his words were for this man only, Amir said, "Father, I want you to know that I will make you proud, as Asif did. I will seek and destroy the infidels wherever they are and strengthen the caliphate. I shall carry on for you, Asif, and the Tribal Cabinet. You will not be disappointed." He bent down and hugged the man, feeling the sharpness of the skeletal shoulder blades.

Amir left the bedroom and wiped his tears before his entourage saw him. Sharing the grief with his father had lightened his stress. He suspected Hasan had understood at least some part of what he had said. He hadn't considered reaching out to his estranged mother. *She'll learn soon enough,* he thought bitterly, *when we plan the funeral.*

As he walked back across the yard, in some respect, Amir thought grimly that the family dynamic and business wouldn't change much because of his brother's death. Amir had always masterminded the attack logistics. He would listen to Tribal Council's proposals and then return with a list of requirements, including how many martyrs and materials would be necessary to make the attacks effective. Once the council had agreed, Asif had provided the materials and training for the attack. Each regional tribal leader would supply the men and women as necessary—but obviously, Amir would have to take up his brother's old role in addition to his own. He doubted he could trust anyone else.

Years ago, shortly after Hasan's two sons had returned home from college in the United States, their attack in Spain had earned them the council's respect as the heirs apparent to Hassan's terrorist legacy. Following a bombing in Barcelona's La Boqueria Market, Asif had led a second-wave attack. Amir had designed the bloody plan and orchestrated its execution. Amir had filmed the mass killing which had aired on television stations across the Arab world. The broadcasts showed images of Asif, praising him as the mastermind. Still, Amir remembered watching with pride, from a safe distance, as over one hundred Spanish casualties mounted.

Asif had relished being the face of the attacks, Amir thought wistfully. He'd also loved working closely with the martyrs and other conspirators to assault their targets. Behind the scene, Amir, strategic and entrepreneurial, had conjured up the complicated plans. But who would replace Asif as the man out front? Duty called—but that was one role Amir did not welcome.

CHAPTER 14

Jaeger stood rigid-faced in the Director's office of the Friedrich-Loeffler Institute. The Director said, "Dr. Brandt, your tenure here at the Friedrich-Loeffler Institute will expire in two years if you cannot get funding and fulfill your publication goals." The short, overweight, balding director, whose rimless glasses perched on his eagle-like nose, went on, "You were a prolific author, but you stopped your productivity."

"You can't abandon me," responded Jaeger. "I must continue my important research! I am too close to a breakthrough."

The Director's face was impassive. "What kind of breakthrough?"

"I'd rather not say because I'm…superstitious. I won't talk about my work until it's complete," Jaeger said firmly.

"You have six months to find funding, or your lab will be closed, and you will have to leave. I can't waste all that research space for you to do nothing."

With eyebrows raised and eyes wide, Jaeger stared at the Director.

"When you were publishing annually in peer-reviewed journals, we could raise money," the Director went on. He gave Jaeger a stern look as he said, "You haven't published one article in the last five years. You have failed to meet our guidelines. Tell me, what is this important work you've been doing in our laboratory?" He asked it with more than a hint of condescension.

Brandt hated this man. Not only was he a Jew, but he also doesn't understand actual research! Jaeger's work was too important to share now with the scientific world. Also, he knew this self-righteous Jew wouldn't be a fan of his agenda.

Avoiding a direct answer, Jaeger pressed his lips together tightly and nodded. He said simply, "Sir, I will get outside funding to continue my work here, where I have been for thirteen years—I might add, ten years longer than you, sir."

The Director's cheeks flushed with anger. "Listen to me, Brandt. My job is to maximize the potential of the scientists who are privileged to work here. Ten years ago, my predecessor and others predicted you would be at the forefront of genetic engineering by now." He looked around his office and then, as if not finding anything of note, asked, "What do you have to show for the last five years of work?"

Jaeger had had enough. "If you'll excuse me," Jaeger said, "I am returning to my lab. I have much to do." Brandt was thinking, *You shall see, Herr Director, what I can do!* Jaeger smirked out of the Director's office, stepping into a quick and precise gait, left, right, left, right.

Jaeger worked nonstop for the next five months. On the last day of October, he took a direct flight from Hamburg to Atlanta, two days before the International Society for Geneticists Conference at Emory University Medical Center. When he arrived at his airport hotel, he registered under an alias and paid in cash for the one night.

He then took a thirty-minute cab ride to the Emory University campus. Inside the cab, he changed into a Halloween costume. As he had read in a university bulletin, he would not be the only one in Halloween attire. Dressed in the mask and costume of Olaf from <u>Frozen</u> and carrying a heavy trick or treat bag, he walked around the campus, trying to seem like a leisurely neighborhood resident. He had memorized the map, locating the largest undergraduate residences. At this late hour, he mingled with hundreds of costumed students walking from one dormitory to the next. In Turman and Holmes residence halls, Jaeger set up two little devices in each entrance lobby. He didn't even have to show an ID. Brandt completed the task, disposed of the costume, and returned to his hotel for a night's sleep.

The travel had exhausted Jaeger, yet he felt exhilarated by his first clinical trial. After breakfast, he checked out of the Airport Hotel and cabbed to the Emory Conference Center to check-in for the symposium.

Two nights later, without the costume, he snuck back into the dorms, furtively removed the four gadgets he had installed, and disposed of them in an off-campus dumpster. If the experiment proved a success, all the victims would die.

Jaeger took pleasure in how straightforward it had all been. But that wasn't enough: he had to learn the details of the outcome. So, he stayed in town as a visiting scholar and attended the end of the week Emory Department of Medicine grand rounds to find out whether his dormitory air fresheners had worked.

Shortly after Jaeger took his seat at the weekly medical rounds, the Chairperson of the Department of Medicine, Dr. David Jones, stood to begin the weekly Medical Grand Rounds. From the front of the large auditorium, he called on Dr. Kathy Kneeland, the new Chief Resident, to present the cases for the discussion. Kneeland was anxious, peering again and again at the notecards in her hands. She described the patients under discussion: their clinical histories, the findings, and the laboratory results. All four patients had similar backgrounds and had shown identical symptoms. At the end of her report, she sat down, relieved to have finished.

Dr. Jones spoke, "Thank you, Dr. Kneeland, for your presentation. In summary, four patients expired from pneumonia with a flu-like syndrome, all with sickle cell trait (SCT), none with sickle cell disease (SCD). Let's first look at the pulmonary process you are describing in these victims. Can you elaborate on the reason four otherwise healthy college students died of the flu?"

Thinking the answer to his question was so obvious, she recited, "Well sir, as you know, um, symptomatic seasonal influenza is Type A or B, and divided further into subtypes based on the Type of H and N antigens in the virus. For example, the most common Type last year was H8 N7. Of course, the original influenza virus was H1N1, which I believe caused a worldwide epidemic in 1918..." Kneeland continued, despite the confused expressions of some in the audience, "Then, the virus spreads by inhalation and coughing. People developed and died from a hemorrhagic pneumonia. The flu vaccine was developed, as well as an antiviral medication, to protect against the flu and treat patients within the first two days of symptoms."

"That's fine, Dr. Kneeland," Jones interrupted, "but what about our four students? They lived in two different dormitories. Did any of the four receive vaccinations last fall?"

"Yes, sir, they all received vaccines from the University Health Service, as did 95% of the student body," Kneeland said breathlessly.

"Were any of the four offered the antiviral medication?"

"No, sir. The students' illnesses had progressed too rapidly to be considered for mitigating treatment. By the time they got to our emergency department, their lungs were failing, requiring respirators to breathe. Their symptoms progressed from coughing to pulmonary failure within twenty-four hours. All of them expired within two days."

A hush fell over the room. Then, Dr. Jones asked, "Has anyone else been admitted to our Emergency Department or identified within our healthcare system with a similar presumptive diagnosis?"

"No, sir, the daily census did not reveal any other patients with flu-like symptoms."

"Dr. Kneeland," said Jones, clearly addressing the audience, "I think we can all agree that this doesn't sound like the seasonal flu."

"No, sir, but it seems notable that all four of them had SCT." Dr. Kneeland looked flustered. She launched back into textbook recitation mode. "In sickle cell disease, we often see interference in splenic function, which predisposes the patient to infection. Maybe these students were more vulnerable to common influenza."

"Yes," Dr. Jones said, "that's true for people with SCD, but the four undergraduates had sickle cell *trait*, the genetic marker, not actual sickle cell disease. *Do those with the trait have the same risks as those with SCD?*"

Staring back at Dr. Jones, Kneeland swallowed, realizing her error. "People with SCT have no greater risk of infection." Intimidated by his tone, she sat down, enervated.

Jones sympathized with her. She's *smart*, he thought to himself, *but she's not thinking*. He realized, for the first time, how scared he was of this new virus.

He continued to address the attentive group, which seemed on edge: "Last year in the United States, influenza killed 80,000 people hospitalized another 700,000. Almost none were young, healthy people. Something different occurred in these unfortunate college students. We couldn't save them."

Jones went on, "The last time a group in their twenties died within days of catching influenza occurred in 1918. Nowadays, the annual mortality numbers from flu have occurred in the elderly and other compromised patients, not twenty-year-old college students! The only thing the dormitory victims had in common was African American heritage, and each carried one chromosome for sickle cell. Why did only they catch this mysterious flu-like illness and no one else? Did they cough and not spread the infection?"

Nobody noticed the buttoned-up German physician who sat in the back of the lecture hall, poker-faced, hiding a smile and an impulse to jump up and cheer. He smiled inwardly to hear of his mission's success.

Brandt looked forward to returning to the Institute, encouraged to produce the subsequent clinical trial. He left the rounds before the next presentation. The lights were low, and he slipped out unnoticed.

CHAPTER 15

After passing by the receptionist in the Institute's front lobby, Dr. Brandt walked to elevator B and rode up to the fourth floor, where his lab was located. He had half the floor to himself.

Jaeger walked to his private office, ignoring the lab's secretary; women in his workplace made him uncomfortable. Since the Institute employed her, she cost him nothing to answer his phones and purchase office supplies. Brandt did all his communications, presentations, and record-keeping. Absolute privacy was essential.

Just inside Brandt's outer door, the secretary sat, ostensibly guarding the three doors behind her. The door with a sign Room 1 led to Brandt's small private office. The second entry, labeled Room 2, his Biosafety Level Four virus storage area, was air sealed and required special suits to enter. The third door, Room 3, opened into the mechanical engineering space. After donning a long, white lab coat, Brandt walked into room three, where his two assistants were working. He approached the lab bench, where they were busy building small metallic gadgets.

A knock at the outer door caused the secretary to rise and open the door. The Institute's Director waddled in.

"Hello, is Dr. Brandt in?" asked the Director.

"Yes, sir, he's in the lab. I'll tell him you are here."

Coming out of the door from room three, his nose raised, and his brow tightened as if he smelled a disgusting odor and looked straight at the Director; Brandt demanded, "What brings you to my laboratory—for the first time, I might add?"

"I wanted to inform you that your funding arrived for the next two years," the Director said without enthusiasm. "Congratulations, Brandt. May I ask you where you received the funding?"

It's none of your business, Jaeger thought to himself. "Several people who heard a presentation of mine supported my work. Their funds flow from a bank in Switzerland, and they prefer to maintain anonymity," he said. He was obligated not to reveal anything else about the Group.

"As the Director, I need to know the funding came from a reputable source," Jaeger's boss persisted. "Who is your donor?"

"I am insulted by your implication, sir. The donor is reputable because I am telling you so. Good day, Herr Director." Brandt returned to the lab, closing the door behind him.

The Director was speechless. There was no way he would let this stand! But then again, Brandt had secured enough funding to continue his work for at least two more years. The Director stumbled as he turned and left in a huff.

The comfort of being inside his laboratory, the success of the second clinical trial in the tropics, along with his anger at his boss, strengthened his determination. He sat at the end of his lab bench, where he often daydreamed about solutions to the problems facing his experiments. His lab assistants knew to leave him alone when he tilted his head up and to the side and entered a dream state. Jaeger was sure he did his best reasoning in those moments. How proud his uncle would have been, he thought, if he had lived to see Jaeger's accomplishments.

Caught up in his reverie, Jaeger hadn't greeted his technicians. He walked over to the two of them working at their bench. "Good morning. How are things going today?" asked Brandt.

Both men pulled back as Bern spoke: "Well, sir, I am sorry to report the progress had been slower than expected. The bacteria reproduction was behind schedule and held everything up."

"Has the temperature in the incubators been stable?"

"Yes, sir," answered Bern. "They are maintaining the correct temperature of 38 degrees Celsius."

"Check the temperature logs on the incubator. Were the temperatures kept exactly at 38, or did they drift? You know the temperatures decreasing two degrees would retard the growth."

"We'll check the logs. Our Cas9 protein production is minimal and not enough to engineer the supply of viruses. Also, the H1N1 growth has slowed as well. I'm not sure why the virus isn't behaving as it did in the beginning."

"Impossible!" Jaeger threw up his hands in frustration. "I leave the lab for a few days, and you screw up everything! Did the two of you check the key parameters every day as I instructed?"

The other technician, Hans, kept his head down and couldn't look Dr. Brandt in the face. Bern answered again, "Yes, sir. Exactly as you instructed."

Jaeger turned to look at the bacterial incubators and the monitors on the virus incubators for himself. Using his ingenious modifications of CRISPR technology for genetic engineering, Jaeger learned how to instruct the virus to destroy a particular tumor cell. If he had continued in this trajectory, curing solid cancers would have been within his reach. But rather than direct his work at a tumor, he had a different target.

Brandt instructed Bern and Hans on slight alterations to speed up the reproduction of both the bacteria and the engineered virus. Then he returned to his private office and closed the door. The slight delay was acceptable if the work product was perfect.

CHAPTER 16

Waiting for the King's Gulfstream 650 to return to Riyadh bearing Asif's body seemed to take forever. Random thoughts raced through Amir's head as he pondered the recent changes in his life. For the Kingdom, his most important job was as Minister for Economics. Amir was glad he had completed the monthly report before Asif's death. At least that was one less thing to worry about.

Amir had a reputation for managing his working relationship with the King and the Prince effectively. His work in this role had taught him that the state's pursuit of Islamic domination was of secondary importance to them; it was not as critical as their oil exports or their status in the world economy. The King delegated all terrorist activities to the Khan family. The royals remained able to express plausible deniability by not knowing any details, despite discreetly financing the family's activities.

It was difficult for Amir to focus on his thoughts with a full platoon of guards waiting nearby for instructions. They would accompany Amir to the airport and facilitate the transfer of his brother's body. Expecting the pilot's call, Amir returned to his private office, where Shazia, his twin sister, was waiting. She asked, "Do you have any details about Asif?"

Shazia, dressed in her typical work dress, a black jilbab, and white headscarf, was sitting in Asif's leather-lined chair. She was attractive in anything she wore— five feet eight inches tall with dark features and an athletic, curvaceous body. She had never sat in Asif's chair before. Amir just stared at her, speechless.

"Shazia, please sit anywhere else. Just not in his seat," Amir asked softly.

Knowing what Amir must have been thinking, her big, sultry eyes just stared at him. Resolute, she said, "Asif died. I lost a brother, too. But we need to move on."

Speaking louder, "His chair shall remain empty, at least for now. That's what I need." He tried to stare her down but couldn't. Amir strode over. "Here, Shazia, allow me to help you," he said as he put his arms under her to lift her to an adjacent chair.

Her eyebrows rose, and her lips parted as she showed her clenched teeth, pointing to the ground. "Put me down, this instant! What are you doing?" she screamed in indignation as he dropped her in the new chair.

His face blank, Amir said, "Asif can no longer sit with me, with us. I miss him."

Shazia, not letting up, answered, "Get over it. He was my brother too." She made a stern face at him. "Given how he bullied you, I would think you'd feel some relief."

He looked up at her, "Have you no feelings? Our brother died; maybe he was even killed…I feel a loss, an emptiness. I miss him. Don't you?"

With a questioning look on her face, she asked, "What do you miss about the bully?"

"I miss our chats in this room when we talked about life, about his adventures, about our future. Asif always sat in that chair. When I close my eyes, I still see him there."

"He didn't show you any respect," Shazia said, but her voice was softer now.

Ignoring her question, Amir went on, "I preferred my role behind the curtain, sitting here with Asif, coming up with the details for our jihadist missions. He was the perfect person to carry out the tasks. And now, I must do both jobs! There isn't anyone else." He put his head down into his hands.

Shazia, understanding her brother's fear, avoided saying anything that would upset him more. She asked instead, "What do you know about how he died?"

"Not much. On the fourth day of their ski trip, Asif didn't come down from the top of the mountain. He was skiing and hit a large tree at the base of a very steep run. His bodyguards were not at his side."

Shocked, she asked, "Not with him? Really? Where were they?"

"It was a difficult situation. None of the guards were skiers. Asif skied on the toughest trails. No one could keep up with him on the slopes."

"What else do you know?"

"It's not reasonable to expect the guards to ski with him. Knowing Asif, he probably preferred to ski alone," answered Amir.

"But what about all the other guards who protect our family. Are they to think failure is an option?"

Amir loved his sister's fiery spirit, her rare combination of passion and clarity. But it would be up to him to determine the fate of Asif's guards. Quietly considering his options, Amir responded, "I will deal with them after the plane lands." The more he thought about what happened, the angrier he became. Amir exclaimed suddenly, "Asif dying that way is ridiculous. It makes little sense."

"What do you mean?" asked Shazia.

"Our brother was a downhill racer because he was tough, fearless, and wild. He once sprained his knee, which was his worse injury. Skiing out of control bad enough to hit a tree at full speed was just not possible. I mean, does that sound to you like something he would do?" Her face softened, she shook her head slowly, and Amir went on, "He didn't have a death wish. Life gave him too much fun!"

Shazia remained pensive. Amir asked her, "What are you thinking?"

After a long moment, her eyes gave in. She smiled and said, "He died doing what he loved. So, in that way, I am happy for him. I pray Allah will forgive him." Face to face, and they sat in silence for a while. She finally exclaimed, "What a fucking waste... to die skiing!"

Looking into Amir's eyes, Shazia walked over to him, took him by the hand, and sat together on the couch. Turning to Amir and placing her arm around him, she asked, "Do you think he was aware —of us?"

"I am not sure," Amir responded. "Asif might have said something to me if it had bothered him. He tried to entice me to join his soirées. But it's not as if he had ever found the right woman to marry. In that way, he was the same as us."

Shazia ran her fingers through her brother's hair as she stared into his dark eyes. "Let's not go there now," she whispered. Sitting up, she looked at him differently. Facing him eye to eye, "How do you plan to proceed with Asif gone? It'll be different for you. How do you think the Cabinet will react? Will they support you?"

Not liking the tone of her comment, Amir jumped up suddenly. "You don't think I can be the man without Asif doing the dirty work?" he demanded, raising his voice. "You don't think I'm strong enough?"

"I'm sure you can do anything, my sweetheart," Shazia said, taking his hand gently and trying to get him to sit back down. "I meant... you know, Asif has always been out front, being the fighter, engaging martyrs and followers to support the jihad. You know what I mean," she said. "He was cold, without remorse." She squeezed his hand. "You are more sensitive."

"What you refer to as *sensitivity*," Amir answered touchily, "is my *awareness*. Asif was the proverbial bull in a china shop, not seeing anything around him as he raced through. I'd be aware of all the delicate porcelains around me as I ran through the shop, but I wouldn't care if all the fragile pieces broke. I would remove anything and anyone that stood between me and my goal." He had to convince Shazia and himself.

"I understand," said Shazia. "If our father were of sound mind, he would bless you now to continue our family's work. Besides being the master strategist, you will become the face of jihad. This is Allah's blessing."

Amir kissed her. She knew him best. As fraternal twins, they had come into the world together, Shazia first. As adults, to legitimize their relationship, Amir would have married her if he could have. Of course, their religion forbade their sin, not to mention their parents and all of Riyadh society.

"It won't be a problem for me," answered a quieter Amir. But then, after a moment, he said, "I never considered the possibility of Asif's death. I thought we would go on for a long time."

Shazia got up from the couch, hugged her twin brother, and said, "Call me when the plane arrives. I'll have the pathologists notify us when they complete the autopsy. I'm going back to my lab to finish a few things."

CHAPTER 17

Jaeger couldn't wait to show the Group the return on their investment. Hardly believing his luck, a wide smile covered his face that these four men had come along at just the right time to fund his work. And he expected that, after the upcoming meeting, the mysterious industrialists would contribute more to fuel his unique research.

As he reviewed the presentation on his laptop, he ruminated about his childhood in Berlin, as he often did. Death had always fascinated Jaeger. He was ten when his middle-class father died of leukemia. His mother did her best to raise her only child, but he never fit in with his classmates. The teachers described him as a brilliant loner. He earned top grades but didn't socialize. The other kids called him "nerd" or the "weirdo" behind his back. Jaeger consoled himself with the belief that they were lesser people.

Even back then, as a child, he had wondered what it would be like to end a life. Once, while attending his Grundschule at age eleven, Jaeger got into a fight on the playground with a smaller eight-year-old boy. Jaeger pushed the boy down on the ground, calling him a Jew bastard, making fun of the thick glasses he wore on his large, hooked nose. On top of the smaller boy, his knees straddling the boy's arms keeping him defenseless,

Jaeger pummeled the boy's face with his fists. He continued the assault despite classmates imploring him to stop. The memory made Jaeger slightly wistful. *What was that boy's name? It sounded Jewish…Greenburg? or something-burg? Whatever.*

He remembered how the boy had lain motionless on the ground, unconscious. The teachers had pulled Jaeger off him, then rushed the beaten child to a hospital. He had never returned to the school. After the battering, no other student spoke to Jaeger or even came close to him.

Although the school should have expelled Brandt, the headmaster learned his father had recently died of leukemia. The school treated Jaeger, an otherwise excellent student, sympathetically. Less concern was extended to the unconscious Jewish boy who lay on the ground.

Whatever else one could say about Jaeger, he certainly was productive. Throughout his career, Jaeger had worked diligently, making significant breakthroughs in viral engineering. The Institute's Director believed that Jaeger's work focused on curing cancer. In the beginning, this had been true. Dr. Brandt had discovered how to tinker with a virus to make it attack a specific tumor by incorporating the tumor's genetic material.

Jaeger looked out the window of his office in the Institute and thought how good it felt to be back among the trees in his native landscape of northern Germany. But it gnawed at him how childhood memories frequently surfaced in his mind. He had resented history class, where the teachers talked about how Germany had lost World War II. The world's attempts to punish Germany for nearly creating a pure Aryan nation had outraged him. Uncle Franz, his mother's brother, had devoted his life to preserving the Aryan race. Franz, who had not spoken to Jaeger's mother since before the war, had shocked her by leaving all his assets to her when he passed away. When his mother died, Jaeger became the beneficiary of Franz's estate.

Jaeger had never met Uncle Franz but found his legacy endlessly intriguing. He detested the way his mother spoke of her late brother as the "crazy Nazi." What was so wrong with using all of one's energy and talents to pursue one's goal: a Germany for the German people? Franz's private files and memorabilia appeared at Jaeger's home after the funeral. Jaeger's mother had accepted Franz's personal effects and asked the movers to deposit the eighteen sealed, numbered boxes into their attic.

In the wake of his father's premature death, Jaeger, feeling abandoned, sought refuge in the attic. There, he discovered, in his uncle's sealed boxes, a world he never knew. Unbeknownst to his mother, Jaeger gained access to his uncle's medical legacy and secret Austrian bank accounts.

The files nourished Jaeger's desire to restore Germany to its pre-war grandeur. Brandt read his uncle's first-hand accounts of his research at the Loeffler Institute in the 1930s, including medical studies on Jewish twins. Franz's references to the writings of the American Charles Davenport and the German eugenicist Eugen Fischer gave rise to his enthusiasm for racial hygiene, which Hitler had embraced. Working with like-minded colleagues, Franz had set out to assure the supremacy of the Aryan race. After the war, when the allies had prosecuted twenty Nazi doctors at Nuremberg, Mengele, Uncle Franz, and others had escaped.

The more deeply Jaeger delved into Franz's files, the more he realized that the victors of World War II had written European history. Those British and American authors had no sympathy for the Fatherland.

Dr. Brandt knew that, with modern biotechnology, he could deliver where Uncle Franz and Hitler's Third Reich had failed. Years ago, in his mother's attic in their Berlin home, he had promised himself to complete his uncle's work. He was ready to make the Group's dream for Europe come true.

CHAPTER 18

The Gulfstream 650 had completed its 12,379 km flight to Riyadh. Despite the swiftness of the world's fastest private jet, able to reach a cruising speed of 0.9 Mach, the trip had required eighteen hours of flight from Colorado and three stops. A hot, cloudless Tuesday morning greeted the tired pilots and passengers. Inside an enormous private hangar, the plane's doors opened, and steps folded out. The passengers climbed out, appreciating the warm, dry climate. It was good to be home.

A large black van met the plane. Under Amir's direction, Isam and Jibran and four more of Amir's guards lifted the sizable casket containing Asif's body out from the plane's cargo hatch and into the van for transport to Riyadh's premier hospital. Isam and Jibran never took their hands off the casket during the transfer. In time, the public would learn that Asif Ibn Khan, son of Hasan Ibn Khan, had died a martyr for the cause of Wahhabi Islamic supremacy. Of course, no one spoke of the ski trip, the cocaine, or the mysterious crash.

Amir kept the casket in view from the moment of its arrival in the hangar, during transport to the hospital, and even in the elevator down to the pathology department. The assistants in the morgue opened the casket and lifted the chilled, black body bag onto the cold steel autopsy table. The pathologist cut the bag open, and a foul stench filled the room. Amir did all he could to keep standing as his head dripped beads of sweat and dizziness exploded through him. Clenching his teeth and closing his eyes, he fought the sense that he might faint.

It was the ultimate humiliation, Amir thought, to see Asif lying dead in his shit. He glanced at his brother, then looked away, then finally stared at his dead brother on the pathologist's table, not recognizing Asif's broken face. Tears came to his eyes. Anger replaced nausea. Squeezing his facial muscles, he clenched both fists as he looked into his brother's dead eyes, thinking, *I will kill whoever did this.*

Amir returned to his richly furnished private office on the top floor of one of the Khan family's buildings. The walls tastefully covered with a wallpaper of woven threads and tapestries from Saudi villages. Several paintings of the royal family adorned the room. Amir turned his attention to the laptop his brother's bodyguards had handed him at the airport.

Asif had chosen an easy password which Amir had figured out on the second try. He opened the laptop and first studied Asif's calendar. The schedule reminded Amir of the meeting tomorrow in Germany. Amir recalled the invitation, delivered by a trusted low-level Egyptian diplomat, to attend a small gathering of like-minded individuals to explore possible collaboration. The plan had been for Asif to participate on his way back from his ski vacation.

In one of their last conversations, Asif had wondered aloud about meeting with a bunch of Europeans. He had been confident the hosts didn't share the same dream of an intercontinental caliphate, so why should they use his family's network? Nothing about the collaboration seemed attractive to Amir. Still, he respected the go-between and felt that, if the Europeans had welcomed his family, at least he ought to show up in Asif's place. Amir realized he hadn't cleared the idea with the cabinet but figured he'd tell them after the funeral.

As he stared at the empty chair where Asif had sat across from him so many times, the enormity of what his family had accomplished over the past decades gave him perspective. For years, Hasan had exported loyal troops internationally to aid in the cause of jihad. When Osama bin Laden had sought support for his 9/11 plan, he had depended on a group of martyrs trained to fly 747's into American targets. The Khan family had financed and arranged the flight lessons in the United States for the Saudi citizens. Hasan had also managed terrorist attacks across the Middle East. He had a tight, trusted group of conspirators, which meant a higher percentage of successful missions.

Amir was proud of how, after a generation of attacks funded and directed by their father, he and his brother had expanded the impact of their network. Modern social media now provided sophisticated delivery of their ideology. With the cabinet's approval, Amir could start a plan on Monday morning to attack a remote American military outpost in northern Afghanistan, fund it, provide the martyrs and the explosives by Thursday, and strike the location on Friday of the same week. The Khan family purveyed the tools of their trade wherever Sunni Islamists battled infidels. On certain weeks, he had arranged multiple attacks in different countries. Thanks to the brothers' hard work, The PLO, Hamas, and the Taliban Sunni Islamists depended on the Khan family for support.

Staring at Asif's empty chair, Amir thought back to the Cabinet's greatest triumph: the attack by homegrown Spanish Muslims in a densely populated marketplace in Barcelona.

Whatever qualms he had about his late brother's character; Amir had to admit that the two of them had shared a calling. During the month of preparations for the attack in Spain, Asif recruited the men and provided technical instruction on guns, grenades, and bombs. Having masterminded the logistics, Amir communicated the last-minute details from 400 meters away. They had been a great team, he thought wistfully.

Two days after the La Boqueria slaughter, seated in their lavish office where Amir now sat alone, Asif had shown him the front-page headline of El Pais, Spain's largest daily newspaper: "Muslim Extremists Slaughter 200 Morning Shoppers." He kept a copy of the paper opened to the full-page photos of the bombed-out small shops. Even now, thinking back to that day, the successful attack motivated Amir to work on a grander scale. What if he could arrange attacks simultaneously in multiple major cities across Europe and America?

America seemed to be the next frontier of the Wahhab mission. In the last twenty years, the population of Muslims in the United States had grown. The diversity of the Muslim community made it easier for the cells loyal to the Khan family to go undetected. With a growing base of believers, the source for martyrs grew, and attacks —Amir trusted— would follow.

His father's work on 9/11 had heralded a new era-—but there was still a great deal of work ahead. *No one could deny*, Amir thought with some pride, *that 9/11 had changed America forever.* Muslims around the world, and Sunnis in particular, still did not control their destiny.

This thought gave Amir a new feeling of resolve. He needed to get a message to followers of Allah: the day was coming when the West would have no choice but to recognize the power of the caliphate. He looked at the empty chair and mentally promised his brother, *I'll do it for you.*

CHAPTER 19

The 6:00 a.m. non-stop flight from Boston delivered Max to warm, tropical St Thomas just before 10:00. Pulling his carry-on behind him, he took a cab to the upscale boutique hotel where David had stayed. Walking into the large Art Deco-style reception area, Max appreciated the small spray of floral scent arising from the motion-sensitive air fresheners placed around the lobby. The place looked straight out of the 1920s with a black-and-white checkerboard floor and perfect restorations of vintage tables and chairs filling a spacious sitting area. Around the lobby guests, enjoyed their morning coffee or tea.

"Hello," Max said to the beautiful woman standing at the marvelously glitzy counter with chrome-lined edges. "You have a very classy hotel. May I speak to the manager?"

The tall, thin woman had ebony black skin and wore a loose-fitting blouse and long skirt, her dark black hair wrapped tightly in a bun. She stood up straighter and responded in her native Virgin Island English accent, "Sir, *I* am the day manager; the regular receptionist is on break. What may I do for you?"

Max nodded in acknowledgment. "I apologize, but it's somewhat urgent. My friend died here two days ago in his sleep. His family asked me to facilitate the body's return to his hometown and retrieve his personal effects. My name is Max Dent, and here is the paperwork from the deceased's brother, permitting me to collect his things."

Examining the paperwork, the manager said, "Yes, sir, this seems all in order. The police have already been through there and removed the body. I don't see why you can't go up there to remove his possessions. I'll get you a few bags to carry out his things." Reaching behind herself, the manager retrieved the key. "This is for his room, number 306, on the third floor."

In a minute, the regular receptionist returned to her position behind the counter. The manager led Max to retrieve a few shopping bags. She opened the storage area, a six-foot-square, eight feet high closet. It contained fallen stacks of boxes of paper towels, tissues, and supplies for the lobby. Max noticed that three round canisters made of light brown plastic in the middle of the closet floor, as if they were thrown in.

To the right was a clutter of shopping bags with the hotel's logo on the side. "Someone left this closet a mess," the manager said as she placed the three round canisters to the side. As she moved the canisters, a vanilla fragrance filled the closet. "Here are some plastic gloves and two sizeable bags for you to carry out the stuff you find in Mr. Springs's room. If you need more, ask the receptionist to fetch some."

"Thank you for your help, ma'am," said Max as she directed him to the elevator and returned to her office.

Max went upstairs and opened room number 306, a modest-sized room with one king-size bed up against the windowless wall on the left. The corner room was filled with sunlight from the two windows. A small chest of drawers stood on the right side of one window. On the far side of the bed, against the wall, sat a cushioned chair piled with worn clothes. David's watch and ring, a gift from his ex-partner, Marshall, rested on the bedside table on the near side of the bed. Max sat down on the unmade bed. Tears welled up in his eyes, thinking of how no one had gotten to say goodbye to David.

He said out loud to no one, "So that's all that's left."

There were unworn clothes in the top two drawers and a dopp kit and bathing suit hanging in the bathroom. The closet was empty. Looking around the room, Max admired how few belongings David needed to travel. He had lived simply and modestly. Similarly, in the operating room, Nurse Springs had performed efficiently, using only minimal resources to get the job done. Max glanced around the unmade bed and saw dried bloodstains on the sheets near the pillow. In the pile of clothes on the chair was David's long-sleeved T-shirt with scattered bloodstains on the sleeve at the bend of the elbow.

In David's bathroom above the sink sat one bottle of long blue capsules Max didn't recognize. Around the sink, and on the floor at the toilet base were red patches of dried blood. The box of tissues had blood stains as well. The bathroom's wastebasket contained tissues with blood-stained dried mucus. What did this mean? *If this was David's blood, he must have been coughing or sneezing bloody mucus. David had probably died in his sleep,* Max thought, because the hotel had reported that he was found dead in his bed on Sunday morning. With gloves on, Max placed David's blood-stained clothes in the two plastic bags and the rest of the possessions in the soft carry-on on the floor.

Max got out of the elevator in the lobby with David's belongings and was struck once more by the citrusy, floral scent of the main reception area. Leaving the stuffed bags at the reception desk, he noticed two casually dressed, muscular Caucasian men with crew cuts sitting upright in lobby chairs. Their heads moved side to side as they scanned everyone in the lobby. Apparently, in their mid-thirties, they also looked younger than the rest of the clientele. Max readily identified hired muscle but wondered, *Why here?*

At the front of the lobby, two police officers, standing, interviewed guests one at a time. As Max approached, the day manager caught his eye. Max walked over to her and said, "Thank you again for your help earlier. Which one of those officers is the ranking officer?"

Pointing, the manager answered, "The taller one on the right."

Smiling at her, Max nodded his appreciation.

Max went up to the officer, "Excuse me, sir. I understand you are in charge?"

The St. Thomas police officer, in his well-fitting uniform and polished shoes, did not smile. He looked Max up and down and answered, "I am. May I help you?" Max liked the rhythm of his Virgin Island English.

"I was a close friend of David Springs, who was found dead here two days ago, in room 306. I'm here to identify the body so we can ship him home for burial," said Max. "Here is the paperwork from the family giving me permission to deal with his affairs."

The officer was taller than Max and with the same brawny build. He stared with an emotionless face directly into Max's eyes. He said, "We sent him with the bodies of the other gay dudes to the Schneider Regional Morgue."

Max froze but maintained a soft smile. "Intending no disrespect, sir, what do you mean by, 'the bodies of the other gay dudes?'" asked Max.

"I guess you haven't heard. Two days ago, we found four men dead in bed in their rooms."

Max's face lit up, and his eyes widened, "I didn't realize that. So that's why you have been investigating. How do you know they were gay?" asked Max.

"This hotel has been a favorite destination for two populations: the gay population and the elderly. Both groups have always been welcomed and comfortable visiting our island. I'm guessing that since none of the men who died were elderly, they were probably gay. If you'll excuse me," said the police chief as he moved over to interview the next person.

But how many guests were in the hotel last night? Max wondered to himself. He went over to the day manager again, who was about to enter a back office.

"Excuse me, may I ask you one other question?" Her lips pursed, and her mouth curled downward: Max could see she wanted to say no, but he persisted. "If this is not public information, I understand, but how many guest rooms do you have in this hotel?"

"We have only thirty guest rooms, with a maximum capacity of sixty guests. It has been running about 65% capacity as we near the end of the busy season. With the death of the four men and another sent to the hospital Sunday," the manager looked down and held her hands to her face, as she shook her head from side to side, "I doubt we will remain a favored destination for much longer." She regained her composure, lifted her head, and said, "Unless there is something else, I can help you with, sir, I need to return to my work. Have a nice day."

Max had known, of course, that David was gay. But if four men had died on one night in this hotel, and all of them were gay, that was not a coincidence. *And another man was taken to the hospital*, Max reminded himself. A differential diagnosis ran through his head. Which infectious diseases or other etiologies could have affected the five men? If only twenty rooms had one or two guests, there were probably twenty to thirty guests, of whom five had gotten sick, and four had died. And only men had died, no women.

Something was not right here that he would need to understand. But first, he'd have to deal with David's body. Max left the hotel and grabbed a cab to the Schneider Regional Medical Center in St. Thomas.

CHAPTER 20

Although a contemporary-looking one-story hospital building on the outside, the clinics at Schneider were oversubscribed, with people standing and sitting in lines out the door. Max made his way down the hallways lined with worn, white stucco to the morgue in the basement. He introduced himself to the secretary in the Department of Pathology, handing her the paperwork David's brother had provided. After he had waited for ten minutes, a short, thin black man in surgical scrubs greeted Max in the waiting room with the papers in hand.

Looking at the paperwork, he said, "Hello, Dr. Max, I am Josiah, the diener for the morgue. Please follow me."

Max followed Josiah through two sets of doors into a room that contained a large, boxy steel structure with eight steel doors, four above four. As Max could tell, this morgue was a stand-alone refrigerated unit, with each door opening to a sliding steel slab cooling a body. The cold air and the smell of death reminded Max of his evenings in the anatomy lab in medical school. This dreary place had dulled grey tiles covering the walls and a concrete floor that conducted coldness through Max's shoes. To one side stood an empty steel autopsy table.

Before he did anything else, Max said, "This is for you, Josiah. Thank you for helping me," as he slipped a $20 bill to Josiah shaking his hand. "May I have a mask and long gloves to wear?"

Josiah smiled, "Thank you, sir," he said. He pocketed the money and gave Max a mask and gloves. Walking over to the small square steel doors, he opened one and slid out a long tray that held nurse Springs. Josiah and Max together lifted the sheet to reveal David's pale face.

With teary eyes, Max stared down at David's face. "That is David Springs. Thank you," Max whispered, noticing the dried blood on David's face. More loudly, he added, "Would it be okay if I just examined the body before I leave?" Josiah looked quizzical. "As you can see in the paperwork, I'm a surgeon. Strangely, he died from no obvious cause. David had been completely healthy."

With Josiah's help, Max removed the sheet. Immediately Max noticed dried bloody mucus in his nostrils and around his mouth, bloodstains covering the front of his shirt, the bend of the elbow, and the back of his hands. Max deduced that, *David hadn't had the time or the strength to clean and undress for bed on the last night of his life.*

"Josiah, I have a big favor to ask you. Are the bodies of the other three people who died here in this morgue?"

"Well, we got six people who died that night," said Josiah.

"But the policeman at the hotel told me that there were three others from the hotel?"

"Four guests came from the hotel, all white guys from out of town. But two St. Thomians who had worked there died. They're here too," responded Josiah. "Almost filled the spaces we have. You probably heard that another patient from the hotel arrived upstairs on Sunday. He's in ICU. From what I hear, he will be down here soon."

"Could I just take a quick view of the bodies you have here before I leave?" Max wondered if all six bodies and the guy in the ICU had the same problem.

"You don't have permission to view any other bodies, sir," Josiah said. They stood there awkwardly for a moment, and then the diener added, "But if we mistakenly opened the wrong doors to find the one you are approved to see, that would just be an innocent mistake." He gave Max a wink.

Josiah opened the refrigerator doors, one at a time, containing the other hotel guests and the two St Thomas locals. Quickly perusing the mouth, nose, and clothes of each body confirmed precisely the same findings of dried blood in their orifices and staining their clothes. Max had put on disposable gloves before he touched David and the other bodies in the morgue. He put a few extra pairs of gloves in his pocket. Stepping away, Max realized that they all had probably died of the same cause. Something that could act so quickly, like a toxic gas, was at the top of his list of differential diagnoses.

Max requested Josiah wrap David's body in double-sealed bags for transport to Boston. "There might be a communicable disease here," said Max.

Josiah froze immediately, fearing that his own hands were without gloves. He quickly washed his hands and put on a mask and long arm gloves that extended above the elbow.

"Thank you, Dr. Max," said Josiah, appreciating both the advice and a second large tip Max left on the counter for him. Josiah confirmed with Max he would double-bag David's body and have it ready for the early morning flight to Boston. That was fine with Max, as his plane would leave about the same time, and he could be at Logan Airport in Boston when the body arrived.

Having signed the paperwork, Max returned to the outer office and confirmed arrangements. The hospital staff was so overworked that they appreciated Max getting the body out of the hospital. They had five more autopsies to do on the other men, after all. Max assured them that the pathologist at home would do the autopsy and send the results back to the St Thomas hospital.

After greeting David's brother on the phone, Max told him, "I took care of the paperwork here in St. Thomas. David's body is going to be back in Boston tomorrow. I had to promise that our pathologists in Boston would do an autopsy before burial; otherwise, they might have kept David's body there another week waiting to do it."

David's brother spoke through clenched teeth. "Not a chance," he shot back. "I don't think an autopsy is really necessary."

Hearing this forceful displeasure, Max answered in a soft voice, "I understand your reluctance. But I am positive that David would have wanted us to know why he died. I think it is essential." Max heard the other man taking deep breaths on the line, trying to calm himself. "May I ask you a question? Did David have any illnesses that he kept secret?" asked Max.

The extended silence told Max something. Then the brother said, "I guess there is no reason now to keep it a secret. David was an HIV survivor."

So that bottle of blue capsules was David's antiretroviral therapy, Max thought.

The brother continued, "He was one of the lucky guys who got the AZT combo treatment when it was experimental, and then ART for the rest of his life. The disease never progressed or recurred. That was years ago. He has had no sign of disease for at least twenty years. Other than that, nothing else," said David's brother. After a pause, "Dr. Dent," said the brother, "If you think it is critical, I'll go along with getting the autopsy."

"Thank you—and thanks for the information. Maybe it will help us figure out what happened. In the morning, please go over to the hospital's Pathology Department. You will need to sign some paperwork to approve the autopsy. You should contact the funeral home to begin arrangements, and they can notify you when they have received the body. It shouldn't be more than a few days."

Max hung up and considered the new disclosure. He knew that having had HIV years ago could not have caused an illness that manifested the bloody drainage he had seen in David's nostrils and mouth and on his clothes. He also knew that nearly twenty percent of adult males over fifty-five years of age had contracted HIV. Max placed a call to the Chair of the Pathology Department at his hospital.

"Hi Tony, this is Max."

"Hello, Max, how nice to hear your voice. Something I can do for you?"

"Yes, Tony, I need a favor. David Springs, the senior cardiac nurse on our surgical team, died in his sleep while vacationing in St. Thomas. I am now in St. Thomas, retrieving the body for the family. But you see, Tony, something suspicious happened. David was one of six men who died this weekend in the same hotel. They found four dead in their beds and two more from the community. Now the seventh one is dying in an ICU here. The whole thing sounds strange to me. They are doing an investigation here, but I also thought that once David's body gets back to our hospital, you and your team might have a look."

"Oh my gosh," said Tony. "What do you think is going on?"

"I think they died from an acute respiratory illness. Could exposure to toxic gas or a contagion cause this? I was hoping your team could figure this out. The next of kin is his brother, who agreed to the autopsy, and he will be by your department in the morning to sign the paperwork."

"No problem, Max." He chuckled. "Never a dull moment in my work; we like a challenge. I'll take care of it."

"Thanks, Tony," said Max. Max hung up and then, remembering there was still one patient in the ICU, found his way to the stairs to the ICU on the second floor. Not being on staff here in St. Thomas, he had no clout. Just walking into the ICU wouldn't work, and it may be unsafe. Knowing that ICUs are high-pressure environments, he waited outside the door for a nurse to come out for a break.

Max introduced himself to the nurse as she walked away from the ICU and out a door to a small, sun-drenched garden where she lit her cigarette. "Hello," he said "my name is Max Dent. I am a surgeon from the US."

"I know," she responded without missing a beat, "cigarette smoking is bad for my health!"

Max laughed, "Well, that's true, but that isn't what I was about to say."

"What do you want, sir? This is my break time, and I need a break."

"I realize that working in an ICU can be very stressful," said Max.

"Not usually for me! I've been doing this for years. But taking care of this young, otherwise, healthy guy dying with respiratory failure is killing me. He's coughing up bloody phlegm, and I keep suctioning him so he doesn't choke. He came in two days ago, and now he's dying, and there is not a thing we can do about it."

"Was he staying at the Charlotte Hotel?"

She quickly lifted her head, startled, "How did you know?" The nurse looked surprised and a little suspicious. "The hospital was trying to keep that a secret, and I shouldn't be talking about it."

"My friend David died there on Sunday. I just visited him in this hospital's morgue. Five others also died there. Two were hotel employees; the rest were guests at the hotel."

She shook her head. "Something bad is happening there."

Despite having intruded on patient confidentiality, Max continued, "Regarding the man you are caring for, what do the doctors think made him sick?"

She stared at him for a long moment. "Don't you have patient privacy in America?" the nurse asked. "Here in St. Thomas, we don't discuss patient details, and I have already said too much."

Realizing he had gone too far, he backpedaled, "Yes, of course. I apologize for that. You see, my friend David, was our surgical team nurse on my cardiac surgery team. I am desperate to find out what killed them."

The nurse with the cigarette in her mouth suddenly considered things in a completely different light. She hadn't heard of the other deaths. Thinking her information might be helpful, she answered with some hesitancy. "They are not sure what is making my patient so sick. One consultant said it seemed he might have breathed poison gas." She slowly inhaled another long drag on her cigarette, then blew it out and sighed. "They can't rule out infection, but the initial lab results don't suggest bacterial infection.

It's not flu season, and we have seen nothing this bad in my twenty years here. We're giving him everything we have. Still, he has developed an acute respiratory distress syndrome, which is about to kill him

"Sorry, you're having such a hard time with this patient," said Max. "Try to find the satisfaction that you and your team are doing the best that can be done for him. We can't cure everybody. We are only nurses and doctors, not gods." The nurse smiled appreciatively.

Max then returned to the Charlotte Hotel. When he entered the lobby, the police officer in charge of the investigation was still talking with people. The line of hotel guests being interviewed had shrunk to only the two elderly couples. The officer was taking his time with each interview. The two muscular goons were no longer there.

Max retrieved David's bags and sat down in the lobby and looked around. The smell, like a garden of lemon trees, was overpowering. He noticed five motion-sensitive air fresheners spread around. Max thought, *Why so many?* To get a gentle fragrance to permeate throughout, one would think two or maybe three were necessary. Then he remembered the three open canisters in the closet.

Max left the front area and walked over to the storage space. As Max reached for a canister, it expressed a vanilla scent, not a citrus fragrance. He tested the other two, receiving the same vanilla fragrance. The manager was correct. Someone had thrown working air fresheners into the closet. *Strange*, thought Max. He slipped one into the plastic bag with David's clothes and returned to the lobby. He furtively removed one device from the back corner and placed it into the other bag. Max noticed that it was much heavier than the one he had just taken from the closet. He'd put his luggage underneath the plane so he wouldn't have to deal with someone asking questions about the contents.

The following morning, Max arose at 5:00 a.m. to catch the first flight to Boston. The Cyril E. King Airport in the Charlotte Amalie West area of the Island of St. Thomas was a typical Caribbean island airport. There was a single-floor terminal building that serviced arrivals, departures, private jets, and cargo. The runway had no waiting line. After checking his bags, Max walked the length of the red-colored stucco building and then through the opened door with a sign: CARGO AREA. A pleasant officer greeted him and asked if he could help. Max showed him the paperwork for David's body, and together they walked over to the cargo plane headed for Boston, onto which two attendants hoisted the casket.

Max's flight landed at Logan Airport four hours later, a few minutes before the cargo plane. After arranging transport for David's body to the Boston hospital's morgue, Max retrieved his luggage and took a cab to the hospital, so he'd be on time for his 1:00 p.m. surgery. He let out a sigh he hadn't realized he'd been holding in. It was going to be a busy week.

CHAPTER 21

On the same day that Max was retrieving David's body from St. Thomas, Asif's bodyguards, Isam and Jibran, found themselves back in Riyadh for a debriefing. As instructed, the two walked to a basement of a nondescript office building in an undeveloped area five kilometers north of the Khan family compound. Amir waited, seated in the front of a modest darkened room. Soft lights barely lit the space, leaving the back of the room in shadow. Standing around the seated Amir were his four loyal bodyguards, stiff and with intense faces, who stared at Isam and Jibran as the two men entered the room.

The heavy soundproof doors locked behind them with a loud clang. The 500-square-foot room had a ten-foot ceiling and walls covered with sound-insulating panels. Dark black tiles covered the floor. Two black steel tables, surrounded by a handful of folding chairs, stood behind Amir. No security cameras recorded what transpired here.

Jibran and Isam had been in this room before. They thought of it as Asif's room, where he made plans for upcoming attacks. Given what had just happened to their boss, though, they felt uneasy. Would Amir be their new boss?

No one spoke until Amir began, in a calm, controlled voice: "Thank you for bringing my brother home. I want you to recount the activities of the days you spent with my brother on the ski mountain."

Isam spoke first and at length. Jibran just looked at Isam as he recounted each of the four days of skiing in Aspen. After dining, they had slept in the rented house. He recited each day's itinerary: where they had eaten meals, where they had skied, and where they had gone for dinner. Isam omitted the drugs, the drinking, and the women.

Amir suspected the details of his brother's indulgences and did not appreciate Isam's decision to withhold information. Amir, turning to Jibran, asked him directly, "Do you have anything to add?"

Jibran found himself squeezed. If he told the truth, he feared Amir would be ashamed and angry. If he withheld the facts, he protected the integrity of both his deceased boss and his friend Isam. He responded, "I have nothing to add to Isam's words."

Hearing that, Amir stood and approached Jibran and looked him in the eyes. Staring in his face, a foot away, Amir quickly withdrew his knife from the back of his belt, and before Jibran or the others could react, deftly stabbed Jibran through the eye and into the brain. The assault was fatal in seconds. With blood spurting out of the collapsed eyeball, Jibran's body dropped to the floor.

Amir fought the nausea he felt and sat for a minute. He didn't want to appear weak in front of his men. Taking slow deep breaths, he just stared up at Isam.

Isam's body trembled and sweated. He felt a stream of urine run down the leg of his pants. The hilt of the knife stuck out from the Jibran's eye socket. Isam couldn't bring himself to look. He noted contorted faces on the other four guards.

Calmly, Amir looked up at Isam, "Do you have anything to add to your story?"

Isam's voice quavered, then steadied. "I withheld information out of loyalty to your brother, sir. I wanted to protect his reputation."

Amir forced out, "I want the truth," but he fought worsening dizziness. He shut his eyes so as not to see the room spin. "Go ahead, Isam, continue."

Staring down at the seated Amir directly in front of him, Isam saw the man growing pale, and eyes squeezed shut. He continued, "Sometimes your brother drank too many vodka martinis. Also, each night and morning after the meal, he snorted a strip of white powder—cocaine."

The anger aroused in Amir got his adrenaline going. He had known about Asif's history of drinking, but he hadn't known that Asif used cocaine. Amir grimaced at the thought that his guards knew of this shameful fact.

His head clearing, feeling stronger, Amir said, "Tell me, Isam, how do you know Asif consumed the white powder?"

Isam hesitated, then looked down at Jibran's corpse on the floor, with the hilt of the knife protruding from the eye socket. He shuddered. "Sir, I am complicit. He instructed me to buy the cocaine when in Tangiers on a recent recruiting mission, planning for this ski trip." Isam was trembling but tried not to show it. "Sir, I was a good loyal guard and did whatever your brother instructed. I would never disobey him. If I could, I would have given my life for him." Isam wondered if he should share anymore like Asif had slept with a different woman each night. He wasn't sure Amir knew about that.

This was a mistake. Amir had heard from his brother about Asif's female conquests in the past; Isam's silence made Amir suspect that the bodyguard was still holding back. He couldn't trust him. "Tell me what happened the day my brother died on the slopes," he said coldly.

"As your brother instructed, we rode lifts with him to the point on the mountain where he abandoned us and went up further. We could not ski where he wanted to go. After taking a strip of cocaine, he raced down the same trail he had fallen on the day before. He prided himself on conquering the mountain from the highest point with the steepest terrain. On that day, he climbed to a ridge beyond where the chair lift ended. He insisted on mastering that run before ending our ski trip."

A hint of anger entered Amir's voice. "I don't understand how you could abandon the man and not ski with him at all times. He paid you to protect him! Who else was on that mountain? Did you see anyone follow Asif on the slopes?" Amir knew this was an outrageous question. Isam and Jibran hadn't considered the possibility that someone in Colorado might want to hurt Asif.

Isam found the courage to blurt out, "Your brother lost his life in a ski accident. I know that is terrible. But nothing else happened. I don't understand why you think anything different occurred, sir."

Amir raised his voice, the anger growing inside him. "How could the two of you leave the man you were there to *protect*?"

Isam did not answer; he didn't know how to respond. He looked down at his former partner, dead in a pool of blood, then at the face of his new boss.

Still sitting, Amir slipped a 9-millimeter Sig Sauer from out of his pocket. Without raising his arm, just cocking his wrist, he aimed up from waist level and shot Isam in the chin. The bullet entered Isam's skull and blasted brain tissue out the top of his head. Isam joined his fellow body-guard in a heap on the floor. The shot filled the soundproof room. The four guards, who had spent the last three years with Amir, had never seen him kill anyone. They stiffened up, feeling their stomachs turn. Amir looked at each of their faces as he put his gun back in his pocket. The lesson was effective. "Clean up this mess," he instructed the guards as he walked out.

Amir returned to his office. He had done the right thing, he told himself. He had no choice but to punish such a failure.

There was still more to do. Amir called a contact in Queens, New York, and offered a bounty to identify Asif's murderer. He still could not believe the death had been an accident.

CHAPTER 22

Late the following morning, Manzur, Rhinehart, and two analysts, Tim Jones, and Rahim Shakur, were sitting in a back office at the base lodge on Aspen Mountain looking at surveillance videos. Tim and Rahim couldn't wait to demonstrate the new technology the FBI was evaluating.

"Before you get started," Captain Rhinehart spoke up, "Agent Manzur, here is a copy of the videotape from the hospital of the two men who stole the body. There are several direct shots of their faces, so I am sure you can get an ID on them."

Nodding to Captain Rhinehart, Walid thanked him as he pocketed the DVD.

They connected their laptop computer to the monitor that accessed the videotapes of every skier riding up the chair lifts and skiing down. It covered the entire face of the mountain. Captain Rhinehart said, "There are thousands of skiers on this mountain each day. How are you going to learn anything from these tapes?"

"Glad you asked. We've been trying new, Israeli-created software that identifies images from video over time," responded Special Agent Manzur. "Tim or Rahim could explain it better than I can since they took the course on how to use it."

Rahim nodded at Tim, who explained: "The software performs facial recognition, but it also accounts for many other aspects of people's appearances. Simply put, it singles out and assigns a number to each individual and then follows the one we select as the group moves. Skiers are of different sizes, wear different outfits, and most have their faces covered with goggles or glasses and a helmet. The software looks at thirty-two identifying factors. For example, I can segregate the skiers, by height; the color of their helmet, pants, and parka; whether they wear gloves or mittens; whether they wear goggles or glasses; and so on."

"Although not designed for this use, this could be a perfect application," Rahim added enthusiastically. "The video cameras dispersed over the entire mountain have an incredible resolution, allowing us to enlarge the images transforming a small dot into someone skiing down the hill. We should be able to select out a particular skier and follow them. Using the proximity dynamic, we can identify one skier who follows another."

Agent Manzur followed the analysts, watching them focus on tapes of the day the skier had died. Tim and Rahim took fifteen minutes to find the man in white who had two skiers following him.

"The face in the images with goggles was clearer than the ski patroller's photo," Agent Manzur noticed with satisfaction. Speaking to both of his assistants, he said, "See if you can zoom in on the face." A few minutes later, pointing at the screen, Special Agent Manzur asked, "Are those two skiers following him?"

"Maybe his two friends," Tim said.

Or bodyguards, Manzur was thinking. "See if you can get the faces of those two skiers as well," he said out loud, his face gleefully animated. Once Rahim selected the object of focus, all other skiers greyed out on the computer screen. They watched the victim make his way up the Loge Peak lift without the two other skiers. After getting off the high-speed quad chair, the skier in white hiked up to the top edge of the ridge, then disappeared off the edge of the screen. The two skiers who had been with him must have exited the Exhibition chair and didn't continue onto Loge Peak.

No one followed the skier off the chair and up the hiking trail. Once on the downhill run, he disappeared amid a group of pines.

Walid said, "Let's see that again." They watched the sequence two more times: the skier in white climbed to the ridge and then disappeared.

Thinking out loud, Agent Manzur said, "If no one followed him down the trail, then maybe there was someone already waiting for him. Show me the one hour before the skier in white steps off the lift," he requested. As the two analysts rewound the ski mountain's video machine and then synced it with their laptop, Manzur's mind was racing.

"Find me the best ten skiers who rode up Loge Peak that morning before the skier in white stepped off the lift," he ordered.

It took another thirty minutes before his assistants had something to show him. There had been seven superb skiers earlier that morning. Of the seven, three had worn identical team colors with racing bibs from Tufts University; the other four had sported various color combinations.

Impressed by what he has seen so far, Captain Rhinehart suggested, "Let's forget the ski team and focus on the other four." Over the next five minutes, they saw only three skiing down the mountain after navigating the steeper, densely treed trails.

"Wait a minute," Manzur felt his heart pounding as he jumped up and pointed to the screen, "Where is the fourth guy?" Grasping the sides of his head with both hands, he exclaimed, "How did we lose him?" He thought to himself, *The missing one could be the murderer!* Trying to calm down, Walid said, "Can you find him further down the mountain?"

They reviewed the tapes several times to see if they could find the fourth skier. Unfortunately, he or she had disappeared.

Walid was getting more anxious and felt a surge of adrenaline. Captain Rhinehart spoke first, "Can you just focus on that skier again?" he suggested. "Let's watch him get on and off the gondola."

They watched as the one skier climbed on the lift about fifteen minutes before the victim. After he arrived at the top of the chairlift, he got off, looked back, then climbed up the ridge to go down the steepest of all the trails. The video never showed him exiting the trail.

Ethan had just made it to the back office. "Sorry, I'm late. I had to make morning assignments for our patrol teams."

"No problem," said Special Agent Manzur. "Your timing is perfect." Pointing to the screen at the front of the room, he told Ethan, "Look at the image on the screen of Be One trail. Are there any places to leave the trail?"

Ethan responded, "There are five different exits from that trail." Pointing them out to everyone in the room, he said, "All these exits take you down the mountain."

Manzur turned to Rahim, who was operating the computer, and said, "Show us on a split-screen with Ethan's exits on one side, and the other with all the skiers coming down after the skier in white left the ridge?" asked Manzur.

Everyone focused on the screen. "Are we sure the other three skiers found exits down the mountain?" Captain Rhinehart asked. "Can we review how they got off?" They all watched the rewinds of the other three skiers coming down the mountain. *It was the fourth guy*, Walid thought. *I just knew it!*

Manzur turned back to Ethan. "What if a skier took none of the five exits and didn't go down the trail? What other choices would he have?"

Ethan responded quickly, "Unless he was a magician and disappeared, he'd have to climb back up the trail or go through the woods over deep, unpacked snow to get to the back bowl on the other side of the ridge. That would be quite a hike."

Rahim fast-forwarded the tape until, all at once, Walid jumped out of his seat.

"Look on the right side!" Walid pointed at the screen. "Someone is skiing down, and I don't remember seeing him or her come up." Tim, the analyst, nodded. "Did we miss something?" Walid asked. "Go back to the morning and see if anyone had a white helmet with two blue stripes, a light blue parka, and white pants. I don't remember that skier from the videos we've been studying."

Thirty minutes later, they had reviewed the videotapes of all the skiers from the morning before the skier in white had reached the mountain. Manzur was correct: no one had been wearing those colors.

"Unless he dropped in from a helicopter out of nowhere, that guy changed his outfit on the mountain." Walid couldn't help but sound impressed. "That's our killer!" he exclaimed, then regretted saying it out loud.

The others in the room were dumbfounded. Ethan's eyes widened. He hadn't known they had been looking for a killer.

"I must admit, that was very clever," remarked Captain Rhinehart. "So, how do we find him?"

Manzur responded, "I am sure he is long gone by now. I'll borrow the videotapes from that day—in fact, for the entire week. We'll see if these two encountered each other on the mountain earlier. I suspect the cameras covering the parking lot and the ticket booths would have picked up our suspect without goggles." Walid stood up. "Thank you all," he said, looking directly at Captain Rhinehart and shaking his hand. "We couldn't have done this without your help. Thank you. We'll take it from here."

The three FBI men returned to Denver and continued their study of the tapes. Once they finished, they reviewed the hospital videotape and selected images of the two men who loaded the body into the SUV. Manzur sent quality facial images of the victim, the suspected killer, and the two other men to the FBI's Washington, D. C. office. Then they went out for dinner.

Within an hour of their return to the office, Manzur and his team got a confirmation phone call. "Hello, Wally," said Special Agent Thomas Smith from the FBI's Washington, D.C. section for counterterrorism.

"Hi, Smitty, I am here with our two fabulous FBI analysts who helped identify the skiers with that new Israeli software, Beyond Facial Recognition. So, what did you find out?"

"The photos you sent created a shit storm. The victim was Asif Ibn Khan. He's a known terrorist wanted by Interpol, MI5, and several other foreign agencies. CIA had him on a watch list, but because he was a Saudi and a close friend of the royal family, political pressure made our interest in him a lower priority. The FBI Assistant Director called me immediately after getting off the phone with the CIA. The photos are causing outrage at the NCTC already."

"Were you able to identify the two men who stole his body?" Manzur interrupted.

"We think they are low-level Saudi operatives who probably work for Asif ibn Khan," answered Smitty.

"So, maybe," Manzur was wondering out loud, "they could have been the bodyguards? And who was the other guy on the mountain with him?" Manzur felt his heart racing.

"The other guy," said Smitty slowly, "is a known former Mossad agent, Max Dent. A surgeon in Boston. They thought he had retired from the Mossad. I just emailed you all the identification we have on him. What the fuck is going on there?"

"I think he killed the Khan guy," Walid said. "I don't know how, and we don't have a weapon, a dead body, or other proof—except that this guy, an advanced skier, didn't try to avoid the trees. He was already out of control, probably dying when he hit the trees. The only person possibly near him was this doctor." Manzur was almost breathless with excitement. "I'll run with it from here. I'll go check him out in Boston if that is still his home."

Smitty responded, "Walid, can we speak alone?"

"Ahh, yes, of course." Walid suddenly remembered the analysts listening in the room. He turned to them and said, "Tim and Rahim, could you excuse us, please? Why not take the rest of the day off? Thank you for doing incredible work."

Nodding a thank you to Walid, the analysts left the office.

"I am alone now, Smitty. What gives?"

"Well, Wally," Smitty said, "I need you to understand something. You and I are now officially off the case! They ordered us to let it go. Since there is no corpse, no weapon, no witnesses, and no hard evidence that a crime had been committed, we have been told that the CIA will pursue it."

Indignant, Walid felt his heart race even faster. "Smitty, that's bullshit!" He said it louder than he'd meant to. "They have no right to investigate domestic terror! Besides," he added, "it may be circumstantial, but I can prove who the perpetrator was and that he committed murder. He may be Mossad, but he doesn't have permission to perform assassinations on American soil!"

"Our orders are to cease and desist. My advice is to obey them. It would be crazy to risk your career by deliberately disobeying these orders."

Gritting his teeth in frustration, Walid answered, "Yes, sir." After a moment, he forced himself to say, "Thank you, Smitty," and he hung up. Walid could barely contain the storm of feelings inside him. Steaming, he left the office and went for a walk to calm down. Why were they taking him off the case? He knew more about it than anyone! Manzur still wanted to find this doctor guy and arrest him for murder. And he wanted to ask him a few questions. The more he tried to calm down, the more questions kept filling his mind. He wasn't even sure why this case was so important to him.

CHAPTER 23

Three days after Asif's death, Amir learned from the Saudi pathologist's assessment that most of Asif's injuries had occurred after he died. Vigorous CPR, as performed by a ski patrol, accounted for multiple rib fractures. According to Dr. Ahmed Khalifah, Asif had suffered numerous, tiny impacts to the neck and face and not one significant crushing injury, which one would expect from hitting a tree. The pathologist told Amir that he couldn't explain how skiing into a tree could kill someone immediately without a massive head injury or a broken neck. One observation the pathologist had made was that the wounds on the neck were like shotgun injuries from multiple small projectiles—and yet, there were no metallic pellets found in the neck. Someone had killed his brother. But how?

The inexplicable nature of Asif's death haunted Amir. Presiding over his brother's funeral earlier that day had been the most painful act Amir had performed. Despite Asif's personal failings, Amir had trusted him as he trusted no one else, except their sister. He had always felt safest when Asif and his men were around. But now, Amir had to ensure his own protection. That's why he had had to make an example of Asif's bodyguards. He demanded absolute loyalty from his men. If he wanted respect from those around him, he had to avenge his brother's death. And from his brother's mysterious murderer, he wanted more than respect: he wanted revenge.

Taking a deep breath, Amir focused on addressing Asif's remaining obligations. He knew his brother had had a meeting planned with certain European industrialists, but he didn't trust the infidels. Every European businessperson he'd ever encountered had made him feel unwelcome; why should they be any different? Still, Amir made the phone call to a number Asif had included in his laptop calendar.

"Greetings, sir. My name is Amir Khan, the brother of Asif Khan, whom you had invited to meet with your colleagues. I am calling you from Riyadh, where my brother's body has been returned following—" he paused—, "his accidental death. Tomorrow is the upcoming meeting," Amir finished.

"Thank you for calling," said the voice on the other end of the line. "I am the representative of the men who invited your brother to the meeting. Please accept our condolences on the loss of your brother. But first, we must verify you are who you say you are."

Feeling a little testy, Amir answered, "Look, I don't even know you. I just have a number my brother left behind. Who are you?"

"Our names are not important. I am only a representative. Before I can assist you, please give me some identifying information. Who is your father?"

Withholding his contempt for this arrogant European, Amir answered, "My father's name is Hasan. The representative you sent to meet with Asif sought our family to help with your plan. My brother was told that you were bringing a special guest from Germany with a new weapon. We assumed you wanted us to test it. I called to assure you that you can depend on our cooperation. Of course," Amir's tone took on a slight edge, "if you no longer wish for our participation, we will continue on the path we have followed for two generations without your help."

The representative spoke in a professional tone. If he felt disgusted at having to deal with yet another Arab, he didn't reveal it. This brother impressed him with his eloquence. Yes, this had to be Asif's younger brother, the one who attended Harvard. The representative hoped he'd be more civilized and pleasant to deal with than Asif.

"Forgive me for being so careful," he said politely. "Only a few people have this number. I didn't expect your call and am truly sorry to hear of your brother's passing. We welcome your participation at the next meeting. We will reschedule it for three days hence. I'll send you the details."

The call ended. Amir wouldn't miss an opportunity to intensify and broaden his activities directed at growing the caliphate. He wondered what kind of weapon they were going to share with him. *True,* he thought, *I don't trust these Europeans. They won't stop. Once they've rid themselves of the Jews, the Muslims will be next.* In France alone, Amir knew, Muslims were ten percent of the population and growing. Still, he felt anxious. He feared he would come to regret this alliance.

CHAPTER 24

The cold, constant downpour pushed Max to drive instead of taking his daily morning walk to the hospital to make rounds. The day before, he had performed another four surgeries, and he now had eight post-operative inpatients to visit. Checking on all his patients usually took an hour, but today it was taking longer. Max then went down to the pathology department to speak with Dr. Anthony Di Bona, the Department Chair.

"Hi Max," said Tony. "David Springs's brother came by and signed the paperwork. We'll be starting the autopsy on David around noon. I'll call you when it's done. Do you have specific concerns?"

"Thank you, Tony, for taking this case. I don't know why and how he died. He was fine when he left Boston last Wednesday. Not sure it's relevant, but he was gay and stayed in a hotel where they welcomed the gay population for years. At least five other men died in the same hotel on the same night—I assume they were gay, too, based on what a police officer on the scene told me. The only other thing I know is that David had broken up with his partner about two weeks before that. I worked with him last week, and he was in perfect health."

"Do you have any more information about the other men who died that night?" Tony asked.

"Well, when I identified David's body in the morgue, the other five men also appeared to have been coughing up blood-tinged mucus before they died. In addition, there was one man actively dying in the ICU at the St. Thomas Hospital, also from the same hotel. He was being treated for acute respiratory distress syndrome with a bloody cough. They all seemed to have gotten sick around the same time and in the same way. I'm not sure when each man checked into the hotel. From what I learned, no one else reported sick from that hotel or the other island hotels."

Tony was staring at him fixedly. "And there are no other hospitals on the island?"

"That's correct. But someone could have gone home sick and then died at home."

"I've never heard of anything like this," Tony said. "Anything else I should know?"

"One more thing. David's brother shared with me that he had been an HIV survivor for over twenty years. That may not be in his hospital record. I don't think it was relevant...but I figured I'd mention it."

"We'll keep that in mind. I'll call you when I have completed the autopsy and will notify the funeral home."

"Thank you, Tony."

"Anything for you, Max." Tony winked and flashed him a thumbs-up sign with his hand. "One never knows when one might need heart surgery!"

Thursdays were usually his research days, but he canceled the afternoon lab meeting. The loss of David and the mystery surrounding his death had unnerved him. It was Lilah's day off. Max went home to catch her before she went to the gym to exercise.

The heavy rain was winding down. The icy wind blowing off the harbor chilled the intermittent drizzle. At least it wasn't snow, Max thought. He left the hospital and drove to his condo. As he pulled onto his street, he noticed a Verizon van parked at a fire hydrant directly in front of his building with two olive-skinned bearded men sitting in the front seats. From the garage entrance, Max watched them for a couple of minutes. This did not seem right. Why would the workers be sitting in their illegally parked van, staring straight ahead and not talking? They were not eating lunch. Looking out his back window, he noticed the two men exiting the van. They were not carrying tool kits. Instead, they had their hands in the pockets of their full-length coats.

Max felt a telltale shiver up his neck. He pulled the car in to avoid blocking the entrance and reached into the glove compartment for his IWI Masada pistol. With the gun under his belt at the small of his back, he raced around to the front of the building. Fortunately, there were no other residents around. Watching from behind a bush along the front walk, Max saw the two bearded men enter the building. They approached the steel reception counter, behind which Albert, the concierge, was standing.

They spoke to Albert, who then looked down at the console in front of him and hit a button. The concierge then looked up and responded to them.

As Albert spoke, one of the bearded men looked down at the console and then back up at him. The other bearded man's hand came out of his pocket with a gun and shot the concierge in the chest. As soon as the gun came out, Max raced into the front lobby, kneeled, and shot both men in the head with double taps as they turned toward the door. Max then leaned down behind the counter to see the concierge. There was an entry wound in the upper right side of his chest, below the clavicle. It had missed the heart and major blood vessels, but bloody air was bubbling out of the small-caliber bullet hole. Max put his ear to Albert's chest and could tell right away that he was moving air through his lungs, but the bullet had collapsed the right lung. He could hear blood and air being sucked in by the vacuum of the negative pressure in the chest cavity. The concierge had fallen to the floor on his left side. He looked up in shock to see Dr. Dent bending over him.

"Don't worry, Albert, I'll get you to the hospital and they'll fix you up," said Max.

Struggling to catch his breath, Albert choked out his words in a whisper: "Two guys," he coughed, "shot me. They asked if you were home," catching his breath, "and they shot me!"

Suddenly, Max heard Lilah's voice on the intercom.

"Albert, are you trying to call me?" asked Lilah.

Max pressed the intercom button with the grip of the gun and said calmly, "Lilah, someone shot Albert. I need you to grab my black carry-on at the door and meet me in the parking garage, now! Avoid the front lobby, take the back stairs to the parking lot, and come down in the next sixty seconds. Wear a coat. No time to explain." He then toggled off the console button to his residence so that no unit lights were blinking.

Max then made a call to a certain number. He spoke in Hebrew. "This is Max. Get a clean-up team to my building immediately. Pick up two dead men at the back door, behind a bush, before the police arrive. Also, I need a ride home."

Out of Albert's view, Max dragged both bodies out to the back of the building and hid them behind a bush. One of their coats was used to wipe up the blood and brain matter on the floor and concierge's counter. He called an ambulance to the condo building and realized he needed to erase the tape from the surveillance cameras of the concierge's desk and the back door. The cleanup team, who already monitored his building, would hack the surveillance system, copy the tape, and erase all evidence of what had transpired. Miraculously, no residents came down the elevator or through the front door of the building during this time. Thank goodness it was the middle of a workday.

Max quickly and gently helped Albert to a more comfortable position in the wider portion of the front lobby, closer to the front double door. With more room for the stretcher, the ambulance EMTs could transfer him more easily. He then ran outside to return his gun to the Porsche.

Max greeted Lilah in the parking garage and helped her into the driver's seat. "Lilah," he said breathlessly, "I need your help. Someone shot Albert, and I was the first to find him. I set the car to drive you to 380

Hanscom Drive in Bedford, where Jet Aviation is located. The GPS and auto self-drive will take you there. Just wait for me. I'll be about thirty minutes behind you after I take care of a few things here."

Her eyebrows rose. "Why would anyone shoot Albert?" Lilah looked perplexed. She grasped Max's arm questioningly, looking up into his eyes, "I'd rather wait for you."

"Lilah, I love you. Trust me; this is the safest thing to do. I'll explain when I meet you at the airfield for our trip home." Max kissed her. The self-driving Porsche drove Lilah out of the garage's driveway. All she had to do was fasten her seat belt. Max could hear the ambulance's siren. He was hoping the clean-up team would do their job before the police started looking around.

Lilah found her composure as the car made all the correct turns and stops. She had not seen that fearful look on Max's face before. It had made her uneasy, and *He said we were going home. Did he mean* home *home?*

Max ran back to be at Albert's side before the ambulance arrived. He was kneeling over Albert, who had now passed out but was breathing regularly and had a good pulse. Max suspected he had fainted out of pain and fright, as he probably hadn't suffered significant blood loss. Max compressed the injured right side of Albert's chest, which would seal the leak.

The ambulance pulled up, and two attendants ran out: one pulling a stretcher, the other with an oxygen tank and mask. Max updated them on the concierge's condition and the fact that there was a single bullet hole in the upper right side of Albert's chest. One of the EMTs recognized Dr. Dent as he placed the oxygen mask over Albert's nose and mouth. With Max's guidance, the EMT applied a thick sealing gauze and held it with his hand on the wound. The other started an intravenous to hydrate the patient. Once the IV was running, the three of them carefully lifted Albert onto the stretcher. Max acknowledged they were a capable team. The EMT, who had recognized Dr. Dent, asked, "Would you like to ride with us to the hospital?"

"No thanks, you guys have things under control. It looks like he has a hemopneumothorax and will need a chest tube. He is breathing well enough, so I didn't think I needed to drain his chest now. The trauma team will take good care of him. I'll stay here and speak with the police."

By the time the police arrived twenty minutes later, Max's Mossad clean-up team had removed the bodies from the back of the condo. A police detective started asking questions. Max was confident Albert's story would include the fact that the gunmen had asked about Max's condo, shot Albert, then disappeared. It shouldn't matter, Max told himself, because he expected to be out of the country by the time the police got the chance to question Albert in the hospital. He was glad that Albert couldn't have seen him shoot the two men from where he had been lying behind the counter.

Max introduced himself to the police detective, who asked if he lived there and if he had seen what had happened. Max nodded. "I got home just a few minutes ago," he said. "As I walked up to the front of our condo to pick up our mail, I saw two guys speaking to Albert. One of them shot Albert. As I approached, they ran out the back door."

"Do you have any idea who they were?" asked the detective.

"No. They were running out the door when I arrived."

"Can you describe the two men? How were they dressed? Height, weight, skin color, anything specific?" asked the detective.

"They were thin, about average height, wearing Verizon coveralls. Over there," pointing to the van on the street, "is a Verizon van. Maybe it was theirs? I didn't see their faces, so I didn't get a sense of skin color. The only thing I saw was their backs; they were running out the back door when I opened the front door."

"How well do you know Albert?" The detective was scribbling a note on a pad, furrowing his brow. To Max's relief, he didn't seem very suspicious.

"He has been the concierge since I moved into the building almost three years ago. I know nothing about his personal life. He's always been an excellent concierge and a nice man."

"Did he have any run-ins with any of the residents in your building?" queried the detective.

"None that I know of."

"Do you have any idea why someone would just come in the front door of your building, shoot the concierge, and leave?"

"Not really," said Max, although he was thinking otherwise.

The detective wiped a hand across his sweaty forehead and put the notepad away. "Well, that's all the questions I have right now. We may catch up with you tomorrow for some follow-up questions. Thank you, Dr. Dent."

Max took the elevator up to his condo. He retrieved a few more things. Answering his vibrating cell phone, he asked in Hebrew, "All done?"

"Yes. A Dassault 7X should be at Jet Aviation in less than one hour. We'll transport the two packages home on the plane. Also, we cleaned the videotapes. I assume you're ready for your ride home?" asked the voice.

"Yes, please, but make that a ride for two. Lilah is joining me."

"There's plenty of room," said the now jocular voice, "but you can explain that to Rosh yourself. Safe travels. *Shalom*."

Max took an Uber to the hospital and had a particular car service, owned by a *sayan*, meet him there. The drive to Bedford took twenty-five minutes. During the ride, Max called Shalom to update him.

"Could the two men have been a response to the Aspen assignment?" Shalom asked.

"I don't know, that would be a very fast response. The bodies were sent back to Israel for identification. Maybe then we'll figure it out," Max sighed. "I hate having Rosh disrupt my life in Boston. No more assignments for him."

After a silence, Shalom said, "Max, Rosh is flying you and Lilah home. At least give him the courtesy of meeting with him. He has something else to discuss with you. You can't stop being a kidon."

"Shalom, you are wrong. I can quit," said Max. "I gotta go." He ended the call.

HQ had rushed the plane up from New Jersey's Teterboro Airport to Hanscom. The car's driver pulled up to the entrance.

Max expressed his appreciation to the driver, giving him two one-hundred-dollar bills and saying, "*Shalom, todah rabah.*" As Max got out of the car, he saw Lilah in his Porsche, waiting with the engine running. He stared for a moment at Lilah's sullen face. She was not happy. Max leaned into her window and said, "Lilah, I love you. You're the best!" As he moved to kiss her, she turned away, and he kissed her cheek. *Uh-oh*, he thought.

He sat in the passenger seat and switched the car to manual control. "Let's drive up to the gate." He told her the passcode to punch in, and the gate opened.

Lilah was tremulous as she clutched the steering wheel. She wouldn't tell him she had been shaking for the entire twenty-two-mile ride, fighting the inclination to pull over and cry. Max had insisted she learn how to drive his unique sports car, but she hadn't tried to learn all the modifications. Sitting passively in the driver's seat frustrated her even more. It was just one more reminder that she had no control over what was happening.

"Please make a left after that hangar and drive past the small private plane hangars 'til we get to number eighteen," said Max.

The hangar opened, and Lilah drove the car inside. A man was waiting for them. He directed Lilah where to park. As they got out of the car, Max put his arms around Lilah and gave her a long hug. Her body remained stiff. The man drove them in a four-person ATV to the waiting jet. The plane had arrived earlier and had filled its tanks for the long trip. Leading Lilah by the hand, they climbed the stairs and boarded the plane. A handsome, rugged-looking younger man named Zalman and an equally beautiful, athletic woman named Metukah greeted them in Hebrew as they boarded. This comforted Lilah, but not enough to offset the sense that her world had turned upside down.

"Let me explain why we are flying home," said Max, as Metukah escorted them to soft leather recliners. She served Lilah a glass of Pinot

Noir, her favorite wine, and Max a glass of Johnny Walker Black Label with one ice cube.

Looking at Max intensely, "This better be good," said Lilah.

Over the loudspeaker, they heard in Hebrew, "*Shalom*, this is Captain Romi, your pilot. Please fasten your seatbelts as we taxi for takeoff. We will be airborne in thirty seconds."

Buckling his seatbelt, Max said, "I had canceled my afternoon and came home to surprise you. When I pulled into our driveway, I had noticed a telephone company's van doors open, and two bearded Middle Eastern men got out. The two men walked up to our building's front door and went inside to speak with Albert. They must have asked if I were home? Albert pushed the button labeled with the number of our condo. That was all they wanted to know. One man shot Albert. I came in and neutralized the two—just in time, thank goodness. I called a cleanup crew to remove the bodies."

Lilah raised her eyebrows again but remained unemotional. "What did you do with the bodies?"

Max pointed with his thumb to the back of the plane, and she shuddered. "EMTs in an ambulance took care of Albert and got him to the hospital. He's going to be okay."

"Why would anybody shoot Albert?" Lilah asked again. "And why did they ask for you?"

"They came to kill me," Max said very matter-of-factly.

"Why…" asked Lilah. Before he could answer, she said, "You mean you *killed* them?" Lilah was shaking even more now. "Max, I'm scared," she said tearfully. The plane continued to climb above the afternoon's overcast sky. Lilah turned away from him and looked around.

As the plane leveled off, Max observed Lilah glancing around the upscale private jet. She may have been impressed by the polished wood paneling and the leather reclining seats, but she was still angry with him.

Metukah approached the two passengers. "I suspect that you and Zalman do other things besides staffing this plane?" Lilah asked, noticing an agility and strength in every movement the two made. Lilah was unaware that Max knew both Metukah and Zalman as fellow Mossad agents.

"Sometimes," Metukah said with a mysterious smile. "We'll be serving dinner in thirty minutes. May I get you anything?"

When Metukah walked away, Max said, "Lilah, there are many questions I need to answer, and there's a lot I want to share with you. Once you hear my entire story, you may not like it, but it will be the whole truth. We are going to Israel because I love you. It's safer for you there— and I have a few things to resolve." Lilah was gazing at him, expectant and wary. Her eyes and her silence told him he had better keep talking.

"This all started," he said, "when you were a little girl, as you know, I moved in next door to your family to live with my Aunt Gila. I survived the suicide bombing of my family for a reason. The pact I made with Gila and God was to fulfill my parents' very different visions for me. Their dreams became my compass." Lilah nodded.

"My father wanted me to live a life to preserve and protect Eretz Israel, and my mother wanted me to heal the world, one person at a time, as a physician. As she demonstrated for me over the years as a caring nurse for the neediest populations, she thought the highest form of serving God was *tikkun o'lam*, literally healing the world. What better way than to become a doctor? My father was more practical. He thought that defending Israel from its surrounding enemies was the highest calling. It may sound crazy, but I committed myself to fulfil both of their dreams for me."

"Max, wait," Lilah broke in impatiently. "Sorry, but I already *know* all this. And I know you worked for the Mossad. But I thought you left that life behind when you came to America to become a doctor?" She gave him a stern look. "Are you still Mossad?"

"Living as a physician in Boston did not require my working for the Mossad. It didn't happen that way," answered Max sheepishly. "After a few years here, the Mossad kept me active from time to time. For the years I have been in the US, they've sent me on one or two missions a year, but always in other countries, never on American soil. The targets were enemies of the State of Israel." Max sighed. "About a year ago, they asked me to take on one more mission, this time in Colorado. It was supposed to be a one-off. We spent six months planning a perfect crime, which was supposed to seem like an accident. But apparently, that's not what happened. I don't know how, but friends of the recent victim—I assume — came looking for me and found our apartment. For your safety, I had to get you out of there. Our safest place is Israel."

Lilah was still shaking—not with fear, but with rage. "Max, this happened too fast!" she sputtered. "The cardiac surgeon I fell in love, thinks he is still a Mossad cowboy." She wrung her hands, not looking at him. "Agh!" Lilah groaned. How could I have missed this, thinking, I am pretty good at figuring out people! "You struggled with some dark secrets; but I related them to your family's tragedy. I would never have guessed you were still an assassin." She said it like it was a dirty word.

"I don't understand," Lilah continued, "how anyone can both save people's lives and… end them." She looked at him directly. "Max, there must be much more I don't know about you. This has gone on long enough. I need to know everything."

CHAPTER 25

Max had never tried to speak about himself as he now did with Lilah. He realized he could no longer protect her from the dangerous part of his life.

"What appears as a paradox to you was never a conflict for me, until now," he said. "When I began in the IDF, I was already a master in Krav Maga and other martial arts. I learned those skills as a kid when my family lived in New Jersey, and I continued my training when we returned to Israel. A short time after I joined the IDF, they moved me into the Sayeret Matkal."

Lilah nodded, "Your Aunt Gila told my parents and me some things about you in the IDF, but no details."

"During my first year in the IDF, with a small platoon of soldiers, we made multiple raids across Israel's borders to assassinate militia and Hezbollah leaders who had attacked Israel. Within a year, the Mossad recruited me to apply the same skills on an international scale."

Lilah asked, "What did you do that was so special that the Mossad brought you in after two years in IDF?" But before he could answer, she blurted out, "Gila never shared that with our family. She probably wasn't aware." She leaned in closer, her eyes asking him to continue.

"As a child," he went on, "the idea of assassination by accident I learned from a novel about a fictional Korean martial arts master. He performed political assassinations to appear as natural accidents. That became my tactic in each attack I led for the IDF and the Mossad."

Max recounted to Lilah the first such attack that he had orchestrated during his first year with the Sayeret Matkal, an elite group of IDF fighters. Weekly night attacks were run into Lebanon to knock out gun placements and push back Hezbollah advances. IDF spies learned of a secret meeting to occur in Tyre for the military leaders of Hezbollah, PLO, and Hamas. It was unusual to have all these warring factions meet in one place. Max had planned the attack along with three soldiers, two men, and a woman. They infiltrated into Lebanon, crossed behind enemy lines, and set up an observation post while disguised in traditional Lebanese clothing. The female soldier and one of the men appeared selling tasty lamb shish kabobs from a small cart. One soldier posed as a beggar struggling to walk with crutches, while another dressed as a fruit seller with a small, old pushcart.

The enemy had arranged the meeting at the western edge of the seacoast city of Tyre. In a small field adjacent to the marketplace, the locals constructed a large tent to keep out the scorching summer sun during the rare daytime assembly. Since no one trusted each other, all participants were required to leave their weapons outside the tent. Each leader had his bodyguard standing at the entrance to make sure no one carried their arms inside—but incredibly, no one kept guard over the pile of weapons. In the 105-degree heat, the guards could hardly be expected to remain vigilant.

The night before, Max's team had sprayed the tent with an odorless, highly inflammable agent developed by a kibbutz of scientists northeast of Tel Aviv. Once the meeting began, many nosy people from the marketplace took an interest in the proceedings. The commotion of the guards pushing the townspeople away proved the perfect distraction for the"beggar" on Max's team to remove a delayed explosive device from his pushcart and place it on the bottom shelf of the gun storage shelves. Then, to avoid the expected conflagration, Max and his team ambled away slowly with the crowd of town's people. When his team and the town's people were more than a hundred meters away, the tent exploded in a blazing conflagration after Max detonated the device. Shrapnel from exploding grenades and ammunition killed many of those that escaped from dying of asphyxiation inside the tent.

The effect was extraordinary. Wiping out a large part of the leadership of the enemy militias slowed the constant attacks on Israel for several months. No attribution for the explosion came. None of the militias even publicized the event. They didn't want it to appear as if they'd self-destructed.

"And that," said Max, "was the attack that got me recruited by the Mossad."

"Max, the exploding tent was brilliant. Here I am feeling proud of what you did and feeling the pain of all those men dying in the explosion," said an emotional Lilah.

In a thoughtful tone, Max responded, "I understand. I guess things don't always seem so black and white. Anyway, after several years with Mossad's blessing, I moved to Boston to pursue my medical studies. Occasionally they requested me to orchestrate or perform certain missions for the Mossad. They used a crazy idea I had for limiting Iran's nuclear proliferation. Other agents visited Korea to make it happen."

He told her about another attack which had appeared to be an accidental railway disaster in the town of Ryongchŏn, North Korea, in April or 2004. The train had been carrying several nuclear scientists from Iran and Syria and material critical for the construction of a nuclear device. The event had appeared to the world as an accident—but now Lilah knew better. She just kept shaking her head in disbelief.

"I never let the assignments interfere with my work as a doctor. All my Mossad activities were outside the continental U. S. I kept the two lives geographically separated—until I accepted the Colorado assignment. Colleagues at RAMOW spent six months planning the mission." Max looked down, swallowed, and his face lost its natural smile. He said, "But somehow, I got found out."

"Why did you kill someone in Colorado?" Lilah asked.

"The target, like his father, was a fanatical Saudi terrorist responsible for financing and organizing terrorist attacks throughout the Middle East." Max related the tragic story of the soccer players in Jerusalem as an example of the Khan family's activities. After a pause, he added, "It's likely this man's father financed the bombs for the suicidal attackers who killed my family. That's a coincidence, I suppose, but it made the project personal. For two generations, this family-run organization has been responsible for the deaths of over a thousand Israelis."

"Even so," Max went on, "I didn't want the job because it was in America. A local cell probably sent the two killers. The question is, how did they know it was me? The fact that they targeted me in such a short time reflects their efficiency and sophisticated infrastructure in the U.S." Max let out a breath. "I am so sorry for bringing you into this. I never wanted it to happen this way."

Lilah remained quiet. Tears formed and dripped from her large brown eyes down her adorable cheeks. Max reached over with a tissue to blot them dry. He kissed her and tasted her salty tears.

"Max, you know I worked as a Mossad analyst during my IDF service," Lilah said, struggling to gain a perspective on all she had heard, "and for a few years after that. They had recruited me because I was skilled at reading people. But with you…I've lived with you for almost two years and saw no hint that you continued as a *kidon*."

Confusion filled Lilah's head. Lilah looked out her cabin window, trying to clarify her thoughts. "I am disappointed in myself for thinking that it is even possible for you to stop being who you are. Falling in love with an assassin is not something I would have chosen."

"When I first met you again, as an adult," said Max, "I fell in love with you. Before that, I didn't think I could. Life is so fragile, so ephemeral, that

I didn't want to share my dangerous life with anyone. And now it feels like all my fears about putting you in danger are coming true."

Lilah let out a sigh. "Max, we're *sabras*. We live a complicated life. Never apologize for being who you are. It's just…well, shocking. And I'm shocked I didn't figure it out myself."

"I thought," Max said, "I'd have time to introduce you gradually to my life so you could make a choice. Now, it's too late."

"I have to think about this," she said slowly. "It's no secret that our lives and the life of our country are intertwined. Israel will always be a vulnerable place. Your Aunt Gila often said that it is because of people like you that Israelis awaken in the morning safely with the hope for another day of life." Lilah continued, "But we are living in Boston now. We're both docs who care for patients. What about your patients? Are they less important than Israel? Why take any risk of getting killed and not being able to serve your patients?"

"That's not fair."

"You never talk about how good you are as a heart surgeon," Lilah continued, more adamant now, "but I hear it in the hospital! Nurses and the residents say you are a genius in the operating room. No one can operate like you. You have a gift, Max."

Turning away from her, he closed his eyes and sunk into himself. He was not comfortable receiving compliments, especially after what he had just put Lilah through—was still putting her through. Looking out the plane's window, avoiding Lilah's face, he said, "That has nothing to do with my Mossad work."

"It has *everything* to do with your work for the Mossad. They send you to kill bad people. If you get hurt or killed, you can no longer heal people. What would your mother say if she were here?"

Staring directly into her eyes, Max said, "I think about my parents every day of my life." He sat up more upright. His voice had a sharp edge, "I'm always wondering: If they were alive today, what would they think of me?"

"Max, I am being selfish," Lilah said, reaching for his hand, tears filling her eyes. "I am in love with you, and I don't want to lose you."

"I know, my love," said Max. "I'm glad I finally shared this with you. We are going to figure this out together."

"Max," Lilah asked, "were you afraid I would leave when I learned all this?"

"Would you have?" asked Max.

"I don't know," said Lilah honestly as she averted his gaze. "Right now, I'm physically and emotionally exhausted." She sighed.

Speaking just above a tender whisper, Max said, "Before we make any rash decisions, let's get some rest. Try to sleep. When we arrive, we'll spend a night at our special place in Natanya. The next day I will have to visit HQ. Rosh sent the plane, and I owe him a visit for that alone. Then you should go home to visit your folks. I'll take care of a few things and then visit Aunt Gila. We can meet in Ra'anana."

Requesting another glass of wine, Lilah went on, "You are right that I will feel safer in Israel with you. But I also have a clinic of patients who depend on me. What am I supposed to do about them?"

"I'll help you figure something out. Maybe you could speak by phone weekly to a few of the patients?"

"And the rest of them?"

"Perhaps prioritize the essential cases and tell the others you are on temporary leave."

"But—" Lilah began to speak, then stopped. "Okay," she sighed. "The others will have to live with me being away." She shook her head. "This is going to be very disruptive."

"It would be worse for them if their psychiatrist were dead."

"Max, this isn't funny!" Lilah shot him an angry glare.

"I'm serious. Why not take off a month or two. We could spend time together in Israel, something we have rarely done. For now, please relax your beautiful brown eyes and sleep."

Her tired eyes felt heavier and closed. Lilah thought about how much her life had changed in the last six hours. She was in danger. Her boyfriend was an assassin. And now, she was being asked to place her psychiatry practice on indefinite hold. Were there more surprises to come?

They awakened to sunlight pouring in the Dassault's windows. Bright sun and clear skies were a welcome change from the cold, wet winter air of New England. The two attendants, Zalman and Metukah, approached with freshly brewed hot coffee and a warm croissant.

"Good morning," said Metukah. "There's a kit in the bathroom for you to freshen up with before we land. The flight took longer than expected because of strong headwinds. We should arrive just after 11:00 a.m. in Tel Aviv," said Metukah.

Lilah loved returning home; it always made her emotional. Images of the day before suddenly struck her. It seemed like a long time ago— or better, just a bad dream. She grasped Max's hand and squeezed it to feel the reality of the life they shared. They embraced until the plane landed, stopping on the tarmac at Sde Dov Airbase. Zalman and Metukah escorted them to the passenger exit door and said, "*Shalom.*"

CHAPTER 26

After completing a visit to the FAA office at the airport in Denver, Special Agent Walid Manzur returned to Aspen village. Armed with photos of his suspect in the two different ski outfits, Manzur interviewed anybody who might recognize the mystery skier. Manzur could have delegated this visit to an agent he supervised, but since he was doing this "off the books," he had to handle the legwork himself. He worked the sequence backward, beginning at the ski mountain where the ski passes had been bought. One of the ticket salespeople and the lady in the lunch place at the top of the mountain remembered the handsome skier with a black helmet. No one remembered seeing the man in the photo with the white helmet and blue stripes.

Before coming to Aspen, Manzur had researched conferences that were in Aspen that weekend and learned that a cardiovascular society meeting had been held at the upscale Little Nell Hotel. Showing photos he had made, Walid found several people who remembered Dr. Dent and recognized him as the man in the black-helmeted ski outfit.

Speaking to the bellhop who checked Max into the hotel, he asked, "What do you remember about this doctor?"

"He was very nice and a good tipper," said the bellhop. "I also checked him out of the hotel." The man paused, then corrected himself. "Well, not exactly. He had his suitcases and skis picked up by someone on the morning he checked out."

"How many suitcases did he have?"

"Not sure. Maybe two or three? I remember he had me carry several suitcases but insisted on carrying another one, a carry-on."

"What color was it?"

"Black. All his bags were black, made by some European company."

"Why do you say that?"

"You can just tell those European bags; they're made better and have the fancy combination locks."

Manzur nodded, taking notes. "Tell me about his skis. Were they rentals?" Manzur knew Max hadn't brought the skis to Aspen, or home on the plane, since the videotapes didn't show him checking any.

"No, they were this year's Rossi's. I ski on an older model," answered the bellhop.

"Do you think he purchased those skis here in Aspen?" Walid asked.

"Not possible unless he purchased them before Thanksgiving," the man replied. "The new design has sold out since."

Speaking more to himself than to the bellhop, Manzur muttered, "He must have gotten them somewhere…" He turned his attention back to the man. "Well, if you see anyone else with those skis, call me," he said, offering his card to the bellhop.

Manzur thought that the skis and probably the ski outfits and the extra carry-on might still be in Aspen somewhere. After all, the videos suggested they had not made it onto the plane back to Boston with the doctor. Agent Manzur walked around Aspen and visited all six ski shops, only to find no one had any of the new Rossignol skis in stock. At the bottom of the image of the suspect, which Walid had saved on his phone, the white skis were partly visible. A saleswoman at a ski shop confirmed they were the new model—and that, as the bellhop had said, no Aspen store had any since Thanksgiving. After leaving the last shop, frustrated, Agent Manzur went to a corner Peet's Coffee and sat down to enjoy a cup of hot black coffee and a cinnamon scone. He stared at the photo and wondered what his next steps ought to be. Would he be able to find the skis and the carry-on? He had to solve this murder despite the CIA and his boss ordering him to let it go.

Walid returned to Denver with nothing to show for his efforts. But then, the next day, he got a call from the bellhop.

"I was talking to my roommate, who works at the gondola lift at Aspen Mountain. He also skis on Rossi's." Manzur was patiently waiting for the bellhop to make his point.

The man continued, "Earlier this week, he saw one of the locals skiing on the new Rossi's. They were bright white. He went up to this guy and asked him how he liked the skis."

Walid asked, "Did your roommate know the man?"

"Yeah," said the bellhop. "He's a terrible skier. He works at the hair salon on the west side of town. I think he might be Italian."

Agent Manzur got the bellhop to tell him everything he could about the man. The next day, he visited the only salon on the west side of town. The awning marquee said, "DANI'S." Inside, women hairdressers stood behind each chair. One man strode about like he owned the place. At the end of the workday, Walid entered the salon and introduced himself. "Hello. I am Agent Walid Manzur with the FBI," he said, showing the hairstylist his badge.

Noticing how Dani got agitated and stiffened up, Manzur softened his approach. "You must be Dani," he said. "I am with the Denver office of the FBI. I have only a few questions for you. Is this a good time to have a chat?"

Looking into the agent's face, Dani was visibly frightened. "Sure," he responded.

"What skis do you use?" Walid knew from this guy's reaction he was hiding something.

"I use good American-made K2 skis. I bought them at the start of the season this year."

"Do you own any other skis?"

"No, why?"

"I understand you were skiing on a new set of white Rossignol skis."

How could he have known about the new skis? thought Dani. Then he said quickly, "They are not my skis. I just borrowed them for a day of runs and then gave them back to the owner. I no longer have them." He asked, "Were the skis illegal?"

Manzur didn't answer directly. Instead, he asked, "Where are they now?"

"I don't know. I just left them on my back porch of the shop, and someone picked them up."

"Someone? You mean the owner?" Walid gave Dani a quizzical look. "Whose skis were they, anyway?"

"I don't know the guy. Friend of a friend," Dani said quickly. "My friend asked me to do him a favor." He seemed to realize that this sounded suspicious.

"Was a small piece of luggage also picked up with the skis?"

"No, just the skis," Dani lied, thinking that he was glad that they picked up Max's bag and ski clothes a day earlier. Now Dani wishes he had never used the skis.

"Can I look around your shop?" asked Agent Manzur.

"Do you have a search warrant?" asked Dani.

Agent Manzur just stared at Dani. "If I must get a warrant, I'll turn your whole salon upside down in the middle of one of your busiest days. Your customers will never return. It would be easier for you just to allow me to look around."

The hairstylist led agent Manzur around his shop and opened every door and closet, as Manzur requested. Finding nothing in the shop, Agent Manzur commented, "Those skis may have been worn by a suspect and are material evidence in an investigation. Don't leave the country until you hear from me. Oh, and one more thing: Do you recognize either of these people?" Manzur stared into Dani's eyes as he held up photos of both the victim and the suspect. He looked for any sign of recognition.

Trying to remain as calm as possible, Dani looked at each photo carefully, staring at the two images. Both had ski helmets on. "I don't recognize either person. Maybe without helmets or goggles, I might."

Manzur assumed Mossad connections were functioning here and that Dani was low on the totem pole. He had hit a dead-end for now but felt confident in his theory.

As soon as he was alone again, Dani made a phone call to his Mossad contact. He began with, "Guess who just got a visit from the FBI?"

CHAPTER 27

The Group's private jet delivered Jaeger on Thursday night. The Dassault Falcon retrieved Dr. Jaeger Brandt at the Rostock-Laage Airport, near his home in Greifswald, and brought him to Nuremberg. Excited to visit the city that had heralded the rise of the Nazi regime, he didn't even mind the two-day postponement. A black Mercedes limousine whisked him to the Le Meridien Grand Hotel in Nuremberg's Old Town. Jaeger liked this classy level of travel. He nodded approvingly as he was assisted to the room the Group had booked for him. He deserved it, he told himself.

The next morning, the hotel notified Brandt that the driver would not arrive at his hotel until 7:00 p.m. Jaeger now had the day to revisit the streets of Nuremberg. He avoided the history museums, which were filled with stories of how his motherland had failed in World War II. Instead, he wandered around the vast parade grounds where Hitler had first aroused the crowds to the clarion call of Nazism. Jaeger strode into the Luitpold Arena, where Hitler, Himmler, and Lutze had led the first Nazi Party rallies in1933. Standing in the middle of space four times the size of a football field, Jaeger reenacted the famous walk of the three Nazi Party leaders across the parade grounds. At the end, Jaeger lifted his arm in an extended salute. In his imagination, he could hear the roars of thousands of people chanting the Nazi battle cry repeatedly. He pictured his Uncle Franz marching there alongside Hitler and wished Franz could be here to see what his nephew was about to achieve.

Brandt sat on a bench, and his thoughts drifted back to the first meeting with the Group in Salzburg, Austria, the previous October. Every detail of the meeting lived in his memory. He had never been so intimidated as he waited to enter, listening from the hallway to the introductory remarks.

As he stood in the hallway anteroom, he heard the Group's leader addressing the others. "Welcome, colleagues," his voice was saying. "It is wonderful to meet again in my hometown and pursue our mutual goals for Europe. In a minute," he went on, "you will meet a guest who can speed up the changes we desire. Dr. Jaeger Brandt came to our attention a year ago. He has developed a technology for the ultimate weapon of selective mass annihilation."

At that moment, a guard escorted Jaeger into a large, minimally lit, and sparsely furnished conference room with a fifteen-foot ceiling and directed him to sit in a simple chair set thirty feet back from the table. On the dais in the center of the room stood a large, glass table supported on a cylindrical, blue steel base. Four high-backed leather chairs surrounded the opposite side of the table—and all four faced Jaeger and the screen behind him. He could not discern their shadowed faces because of the blazing backlighting. With bright lights flooding his eyes, he did not see the video cameras recording him, nor much of anything else. His sphincters tightened, not knowing what was next and feeling terrified.

In a perfunctory manner, the leader, speaking in Austrian German, acknowledged Jaeger: "Welcome, Dr. Brandt." Then he continued. "We meet to make a wonderful world, as we push conservative governments to meet our goals, restore the purity of citizenship in our native countries, and promote a return to the traditions that made us once great."

The four men seemed to be looking at a screen behind Jaeger, which he turned to see. It lit up with three words displayed:

CONSERVATISM PURITY TRADITION

The leader continued, "Five years ago, during a lecture at the Loeffler Institute's Annual Public Symposium, Dr. Brandt described a new technology. We learned of this in the past year. I am confident that its application will be of great interest to us. The Group invited Brandt to share his research." He then went on to discuss the technology in considerable detail.

"Is that a fair summary of your scientific progress, Dr. Brandt?" asked Schroeder.

Jaeger breathed an inward sigh of relief to realize that they communicated in German. It thrilled Brandt to hear the man's detailed understanding of his research and echoing Jaeger's private thoughts.

Before Brandt could respond, the leader added, "Dr. Brandt, we appreciate your availability today. The four of us have an interest in restoring the European values neglected over the last seventy-five years. We have a common goal and are prepared to invest significant resources to support that goal. Could you please update us on your scientific investigations?"

Trying to see through the blinding lights, Jaeger felt his heartbeat pound as the four silhouettes stared at him. *Who are they? What have I gotten myself into?* As Jaeger shared the specifics of his work, the men at the table had questions and comments. He did not like being queried by men whose faces he could not see. However, their questions and comments told Jaeger that they seemed to think the same way about the populace of Europe as he did. As the meeting went on, his racing heartbeat slowed, the contracted muscles in his hands relaxed.

One question came from another shadow. Brandt noticed the man had a silky voice nurtured to provide service. He didn't have the bravado or confidence of the leader. Jaeger naturally trusted this voice.

"Dr. Brandt," said the second man with a Swiss accented German, "Much of the funding at the Friedrich-Loeffler Institute comes from us and our friends. Someone we trust delivered the invitation that brought you here. Although your Director, as instructed, passed the sealed invitation to you, he is not aware of us, and he must never know of our existence. I am sure you understand."

They don't trust the Director, Jaeger thought to himself. *Interesting!* "Yes, sir," Brandt said. "I understand and will respect your wishes."

Bernard continued, "You have accomplished much in your field of genetic engineering. Other than what you have published in journal articles, can you share some evidence of a practical application for your work?"

Dr. Brandt was slow to respond. This probably Swiss man seemed gentle, sensitive, and Jaeger wanted to trust him. Yet, he wasn't sure how these men would handle the facts about his first clinical trial. Jaeger had handed a USB flash drive to the guard, and now he turned to see the large projection screen behind him and motioned for his PowerPoint presentation to start. Dr. Brandt discussed six slides over five minutes, providing extensive evidence that his methods worked. He gave the Group a detailed description of everything.

A dead silence followed.

The deep rich melodic voice that spoke next belonged the Frenchman, as Brandt labeled him. "I must say, Dr. Brandt. I'm impressed. But what is a motion-sensitive air freshener?"

Surprised by the elementary question, Jaeger explained.

"Your technology was quite effective," said the fourth voice, this one nasal and almost high pitched, but not loud or forceful. He spoke classic Berlin accented German. "It worked on a small scale. Could it work on a larger scale?"

Now the questions focused on the future, which is where Jaeger wanted the conversation to go. Brandt's sense of trust in these men grew with every question. The conversation continued for another forty minutes. The Austrian leader outlined a series of expectations for Brandt to follow if the Group supported his research at the Institute. With evident enthusiasm, Brandt went on, "I accept those tenets. But, respectfully," Jaeger queried, "I would ask you to tell me more about how the Group works."

This time the man the Frenchman answered, "As you may have noticed, we use no names and conceal our faces. We apologize for the bright lights on your face, which help maintain our anonymity. Our identities must remain unknown even to you. The Group's very existence is a secret. We never socialize with each other beyond these walls."

They shared no more information about themselves, to Jaeger's disappointment. Instead, the Group asked him a few more questions and then thanked Jaeger for coming. Two other men, one tall and skinny and the other very muscular and almost neckless, escorted Jaeger out. When the three reached the outside office, they sat, and the man with no neck spoke.

"Dr. Brandt, thank you for coming. The Group appreciates your time. Your flight home is waiting for you. We checked you out of the hotel and covered the expenses. Here is your suitcase. Also, here is a stipend for your time." The tall man handed him a thick envelope.

Nodding, thinking he was done, "Thank you," Jaeger began when the muscular man spoke again.

"You need to be clear about one thing. This meeting never happened. Only the two of us will communicate with you. You are never to attempt to communicate with the four members of the Group. And they will never contact you directly. One of us will be the connection, either by email, by text, or in person. Is that understood?"

"Yes," replied Jaeger as he felt the heft of the envelope. It exceeded his expenses. Yet he was angry that they had packed up his suitcase without permission. Staring at the wad of cash made it easy to squeeze his mouth shut.

"One more thing: you may not share your knowledge of the Group and everything that transpires in your work with the Group. Is that clear?"

"Yes, sir," replied Jaeger. Brandt was getting more uncomfortable as his head whirled with excitement to pursue his work, but he was also indignant. He had no intention of telling anyone about this! Why all the threats?

"Oh, it may not be necessary to say, but I should mention that any breaking of these rules was punishable by death," no-neck said with an emotionless face.

Jaeger's stomach dropped as he nodded, his guts tight with fear. He told himself he would remain cautious about what he shared with them.

He would never reveal the entire story and all the power of his biological weapon. And meanwhile, the Group had agreed to fund his research for two more years.

CHAPTER 28

A t 7:00 p.m. sharp, the private car drove Jaeger to a contemporary, six-story, glass-enclosed building. The building stood in sharp contrast to the older edifices of the 950-year-old city. The same tall guard from six months earlier greeted Dr. Brandt, without smile or recognition, and accompanied him up to the sixth floor.

At the first meeting in Salzburg, Jaeger had received enough funding to continue his research in the short term. He shared enough details of the clinical trial in Atlanta to earn more support. Today, Dr. Brandt would expand on that presentation with additional slides and outcome data. Hopefully, he would leave having convinced them to fund his work for three more years.

The elevator opened into a large, empty waiting room. Jaeger took a seat as he was told. There were no windows. The room's subdued lighting came from small lamps on the side tables placed at the edges of the large sofa and next to the four upholstered chairs. Unlike at the initial meeting in Salzburg, which had begun promptly, this time he waited two hours in the room, making him testy. Why did they keep him sitting there?

Finally, the door opened, and a dark-skinned, athletic man with sharp features, a small feminine nose, and jet-black hair entered, escorted by a muscular man sporting a crew cut. The new guest wore a business suit and tie and large, dark glasses that intimidated Jaeger. As the burly man began to leave, he turned back and spoke; "Gentlemen, there will be no conversation while waiting here."

The two men's faces showed no reaction. They remained dead silent for another fifteen minutes, not introducing themselves before the greeters returned.

The tall man began by saying, "Welcome, gentlemen. Please follow us into the meeting room. I must ask you to leave your mobile phones and any weapons you have. Before entering the meeting, you will pass through a metal detector and be frisked by two security personnel. I apologize in advance, but this is a compulsory process determined by the Group."

Both men handed in their phones. Besides his cell phone, Jaeger gave the guard a small thumb drive containing his presentation. The other man handed over his two phones, each manufactured by a different company. Jaeger wondered why this mysterious man needed two mobile phones. Who was he?

Jaeger and Amir were escorted into the meeting room and assigned to seats on the concave side of a large, curved table. Behind the convex side of the curved table, on a slightly raised platform, sat four men in dark business suits. Jaeger felt a surge of déjà-vu. From their thickly padded leather chairs, the four men looked down on their two guests. As in the first meeting with the Group Jaeger noticed, with bright backlighting, he could not resolve men's faces at the table.

"Welcome, gentlemen," said the familiar voice of the leader. "Dr. Brandt," who waved, "thank you for returning to meet with us." He turned to his fellow Group members. "You all recall Dr. Jaeger Brandt, an internationally acclaimed research scientist at the Loeffler Institute in Germany. Our other guest is Amir Ibn Khan, the Minister of Economics for Saudi Arabia, and the younger brother of Asif Ibn Khan, who met with us three months ago. In succeeding his father in this critical role, Amir handles the financial management of the Kingdom." He did not elaborate on the details of Amir's organization. "Mr. Khan, we are glad you could make the trip."

The speaker introduced himself as the Chairman of the Group, who Jaeger had labeled the Austrian. Then he announced, "Dr. Brandt is here to update us on his special project. He recently returned from a field test of a new weapon. Dr. Brandt, we are eager to hear your report."

Everyone turned to look at Jaeger as the first slide of his PowerPoint filled the screen behind him. "As the Group learned from me during my previous visit," he began, "I have directed my research to make a virus that kills cells with a specific genetic design."

Dr. Brandt continued to speak for twenty minutes, carefully outlining his scientific work, new discoveries, and recent clinical trial in St. Thomas. Amir listened and wondered who this braggart was. But as he considered the implications of Brandt's work, he couldn't help feeling impressed. The more Jaeger spoke, the more Amir obsessed he had to work with this European. The possibility for selective terrorism of entire communities, with no risk to the terrorist and no need for martyrs was mind boggling. A hundred questions percolated in his head. The Saudi couldn't wait to sit down and speak with Jaeger himself.

Dr. Brandt described the successful second clinical trial. Amir paid rapt attention.

"How did you select this group of people?" asked the soft-talking member of †he Group.

"They had genetic markers that I could easily identify."

"Can you give us examples of other people who you can select for their genetic identity?" asked the Frenchman, whose nationality Brandt assumed.

"About nine months ago, I ran my first clinical trial in Atlanta, preferring to stay outside of Europe until I perfected my techniques. I targeted a genetic marker common in African Americans. My trial was a success."

"By which you mean—" the Frenchman cut in.

"Everyone who was supposed to catch the virus died within twenty-four hours," Jaeger completed his sentence.

The Group cheered in response. Jaeger swelled with pride.

Amir's imagination ran wild. With Brandt's weapon, he could generate attacks on an unprecedented scale. He could wipe out more people than he had ever dreamed, and could do so selectively, without hurting those he wanted to protect!

While Amir was getting inspired, Jaeger was getting carried away. "I can kill all redheads," he boasted. "I can kill Blacks or Jews! Only my resources and time limit my production of viruses. With your support, gentlemen, I can produce enough virus to kill thousands!"

Once he stopped speaking, Jaeger turned to see an unfamiliar image appear on the projection screen behind him, which showed data and some photos.

The Group Chairman spoke, "Before today, we didn't know about your experiment in Atlanta. Congratulations!" Jaeger and Amir saw the Chairman's silhouette turn back to the group. "As previously agreed with Dr. Brandt," he explained, "we sent two observers to the hotel in St. Thomas. Their report raises some questions and contains data and several photos that you have not seen. Our men confirmed the five deaths you described. They also spoke with a man who works inside the pathology department at the hospital. Five Caucasian bodies, as Dr. Brandt described, died from a very aggressive respiratory illness. The pathologists diagnosed severe pneumonia induced by influenza. Their airways that connect the mouth to the lungs were full of thick bloody mucus." The Chairman's voice was full of disgust.

Trying to hold back a shudder, the Austrian used a laser pointer to direct attention to the images on the screen. Everyone could see bloodstained shirts and clothes on the dead bodies and bloody discharge in their nostrils.

Jaeger was concerned. *How did the Group get such access?*

"But two more men died that night who didn't stay at the hotel," the Chairman added.

Immediately, Jaeger froze. *What?*

Photos of black bodies in the morgue appeared on the screen. "These two men also died with an acute respiratory illness and showed the same bloody mucus. Can you explain that Dr. Brandt?" this made the scientist squirm.

"I don't know who those two dead men are or where they came from," Jaeger responded sheepishly.

"Well, *we* do," boasted the Austrian. "These two dead St. Thomas natives were homosexual men in their sixties and worked in the same hotel. One was a porter, the other a hairstylist in the hotel's basement salon. Both were HIV survivors. Their deaths confirm that the test of your virus was a great success, Dr. Brandt. Congratulations!"

Feeling relieved, Jaeger was quiet at first. Then he felt his face break into a smile.

"Thank you, sir. I am ready to begin the next level of virus development."

"There is one loose end, Dr. Brandt," the Chairman cautioned. "As we had agreed, the two observers were to collect the special air fresheners. Unfortunately, they only found four when they returned late Tuesday night to the hotel. Do you know where the fifth one is?"

Jaeger's face turned ashen. Not knowing the answer, Brandt responded, "Maybe somebody threw it out when they found it wasn't expressing any more freshener?"

"We don't have an answer, but we don't like loose ends. Until someone finds out what happened, we still have a problem." The Chairman continued, "We'll set that aside for now as we strategize what's next. Mr. Khan is here to help us with our next steps. The Khan family is a friend from Saudi Arabia. We hoped that his organization would distribute your work product," said the Austrian. "Mr. Khan, do you have any thoughts or suggestions?"

Although he had many questions, Amir didn't show any emotion and remained passive and silent. "No, sir. I have no questions," he answered. His face reflected none of the excitement he was feeling.

"Dr. Brandt, what time frame are you looking at?" the Swiss man asked.

"It depends how much product I need and the circumstances of the dispersal," Jaeger said. He explained that, as in Atlanta and St. Thomas, the victims would need to inhale the virus vapor for it to work. "Releasing the virus in a fine aerosol of water droplets will not work from an airplane at 2000 meters. But I know," Jaeger continued, "that it works if spread at ground level by people just breathing within two meters of the spray. He went on. "It would take my lab three weeks to grow enough to kill 1,000 people in a closed space. I have already created some cultures for specific genetic profiles. With time, "I could develop enough to saturate an area as densely populated as New York City…"

Jaeger knew it was foolish to make promises he could not possibly keep. And yet, having had such brilliant success with the St. Thomas experiment, part of him imagined he really could do it. These powerful men held the best chance of accomplishing his goal: to assure his dream of a pure Germany.

"One more thing," asked the German from Berlin, according to Jaeger. "When the time is right, how do you propose to distribute the gas?"

Twenty seconds of silence passed before Jaeger began to speak. "I believe you are asking, besides the natural spread from one host to the next, how do I plan to infect a large population? I have considered several possibilities but will make a decision once we identify the target population." Jaeger indicated he wasn't ready to discuss dispersal methods, as he continually tried, unsuccessfully, to see the faces of the members of the Group. *Was this response a problem for them?*

"I am going to need more resources to move forward with these plans," Jaeger said bluntly. "I could use more trained technicians and more equipment."

After seeing the nods of the other three members, the Chairman responded, "Thank you, Dr. Brandt. We will arrange more financial support at the Institute. We expect you to work out the logistics for manufacturing and distribution. You should seriously consider working with Mr. Khan on the distribution of your virus. We'll expect your report to the Group for our approval and more financing within three months."

Jaeger's mind gave in as he felt sweat drip from his scalp and hands. His face tightened as his anxiety exploded. The deadline was one thing; working with an Arab was something else. But Brandt wasn't sure he had a choice.

CHAPTER 29

The Mossad's private jet brought Lilah and Max home to Israel. Although Lilah was excited to wake up in her home country, the outpouring of Max's long-kept secrets had overwhelmed her. So much for her professional ability to study people and observe the truths they tried to conceal, she thought. *So, he was keeping secrets from me. How did I miss that?* Had her love for Max blinded her from seeing his double life? *It's difficult to be objective with loved ones.*

Descending the jet's airstair, Lilah stared into Max's eyes and said, "I have work to do with you."

Puzzled, "What do you mean?" asked Max.

"I want to understand you. My head is bursting with a million questions. I need you to set aside time...for us."

Staring straight back at Lilah with wide eyes, Max said earnestly, "Whatever you need, I will make happen."

Lilah said, "Yes, I know you will. I am crazy in love with you," she said, with tears dripping from her eyes, "but I just learned that you are someone else." There was a long pause before Lilah continued. She leaned into him and kissed his lips for a long moment. They clasped hands not speaking until they reached the tarmac and the waiting car.

Like Lilah, Max now had to navigate new territory. He had revealed all his secrets to her. Would their relationship survive? Their return to Israel energized him. Max thought about the Hebrew name of his native country, Israel, meaning "one who struggles with God and self." He told himself, *That's where we are.*

At the small military airfield, the driver picked them up and immediately reached for his cell phone to get his next instructions from Max's boss, the director of the Mossad, whom everyone referred to as "Rosh." Max grabbed his hand. "That won't be necessary. I'll tell you where to go. Then, after you drop us off, you can call it in."

Since the Mossad had sent the plane for them, Max knew Rosh expected them to show up as soon as the plane landed. He sensed that landing at this soon-to-be-closed Sde Dov military airfield had not just been about maintaining secrecy; it was about his boss maintaining control over his movements. But Rosh wouldn't get his way this time. There were few places in Israel to hide from the world's most respected intelligence agency—but Max had one in mind.

The driver dropped them off at the crowded Independence Square in the heart of Natanya, where it would be hard for anyone to follow them. Once the driver had left, Max hailed a taxi to take them to their coastal condo overlooking the Mediterranean Sea. The hideaway contained their clothes and necessary personal items for spontaneous visits. Max had called ahead from the plane to arrange for fresh food, wine, and sundry supplies.

The condo was their private happy place. Max and Lilah kept it a secret, even from Aunt Gila and Lilah's parents. An electric motorcycle with two helmets was maintained by a loyal friend who looked after the apartment and prepared it for their visits. Natanya was a short drive to Mossad headquarters and a twenty-five-minute ride to their neighboring childhood homes in Ra'anana. Regrettably, they had few opportunities to enjoy this slice of Israeli heaven.

It was just past noon when they arrived. Exhausted from travel, they showered together to refresh. Afterward, with Lilah in a pink T-shirt and

Max clad in a towel wrapped around his waist, they drank the chilled rosé from the glasses he had poured. Lilah reheated a French bread topped with oozing brie and placed it on a serving tray with fresh olives on the side. In their living room, the opened sliding glass doors exposed a terrace with a vista of beach, sea, and nothing else. It was March, and no one was in the water. The refreshing sea breeze invited them outdoors. A carved wooden cushioned loveseat drew them out on the terrace where they sat. They sipped the wine and tasted the warm bread and cheese and native olives. Lilah said to Max, "The Mediterranean is so calming. I love this place."

Max put his arm around her and kissed her gently, his lips nibbling hers. He stood with his hands on her waist, and they kissed more deeply. Max slipped his hands from around Lilah's waist and found their way up her T-shirt.

"The sea sets me free," whispered Lilah. The sweetness of Lilah's breath and the sensual feel of naked flesh aroused and connected them. Lilah tilted her head back. Max covered her neck with soft kisses while cupping his hands around her full breasts, his thumb and fingers teasing her nipples. She felt Max's arousal pressing against her.

The thought of Max's double life came back to Lilah, but this time, it didn't faze her. Instead, she felt the body of the man before her—the surgeon, the assassin-—and embraced his courage and his strength.

The terrace sun warmed their yearning bodies. Lilah pulled his towel as she gently caressed his firmness. She held him in her hands and knelt, wanting to satisfy him.

Max closed his eyes as Lilah's affection made him climb. He gently lifted her, and Lilah's legs wrapped around his waist as he carried her into the bedroom. He removed her T-shirt and delicately massaged her favorite frankincense botanical oil into her luscious skin with just his fingertips. The fragrance was as sensual as the feel. Their well-oiled bodies glided over each other's nakedness as they kissed incessantly.

"Slowly," whispered Lilah, as Max moved his soft kisses down her chest, lovingly sucking each aroused nipple. He made his way down her body, caressing, licking her navel, and finally finding his way to her clitoris. Spreading her legs, Lilah moaned, aching to feel Max within her.

Max sensed Lilah's pleasure as he directed his tongue thrusts at her target of arousal. Lilah's back arched into a high bridge as Max lifted her, his hands squeezing her buttocks, his tongue thrusting inside her.

Feeling Lilah climax twice made Max's body tingle with excitement. His hands moved from her buttocks and clasped her hands tightly. Max's thirst for her was insatiable. Lilah pressed herself against his face waiting to explode again in ecstasy. Her scream of pleasure caused Max to feel his body building with an unstoppable excitement. Lilah's body quivered. Her feet flexed, and her toes spread. "Deeper," she groaned as she flattened her back to the bed and guided him into her.

"Deeper," she repeated. On top of Lilah, Max thrust hard as she tightly wrapped her legs around his waist. As Max climaxed, they could not feel more connected, more complete.

In Max's arms, sleep came to Lilah quickly. As his mind drifted, Max smiled at Lilah lying next to him, so beautiful and so peaceful. He had never experienced love as he did with Lilah. Even so, his mind was not at peace. His thoughts drifted to Lilah's vulnerability and his guilt. *How could I have exposed her to such danger?* He thought. He felt a sudden surge of anger at his would-be assassins. How had they struck back against him so quickly--and at his and Lilah's home? *How naïve of me to believe that Lilah would be perfectly safe from my secret life!*

One fundamental question haunted Max: how had someone figured out that the Saudi's death was not an accident? Who had informed the extremist cell that had tracked him down? Worst of all, Max knew his enemies would target him again. It was unacceptable to have involved Lilah. While Lilah slept in bed, Max opened the Johnny Walker Black Label and poured himself a glass. He gulped it down. Whatever Rosh wanted at headquarters would have to wait till Max had had time to think.

As he held the glass between his palms, he reviewed all that had happened. His tightened stomach told him he had to find a resolution. He had assassinated a wanted terrorist, and within three days, someone had tried to kill him—and maybe Lilah, too. And yet, it had seemed like a perfect assassination! He had made it look like an accident. So, who had uncovered the truth and how?

Max's thoughts suddenly swerved in another direction. Why had his surgical nurse, David Springs, died in his sleep, along with five or six other men in that hotel in St. Thomas? Their deaths had been deliberate, but why? Who had managed the stealth attack? And how? Stranger still, before any of this, Rosh had sent him that message to return to Israel. Max felt like a juggler with too many balls in the air. What else didn't he know about?

Watching Lilah sleep peacefully, Max's thoughts turned to Rosh. Seven years ago was the last time he had received an urgent message from his boss. Back then, Israel was under attack from a growing number of rockets launched from Gaza, and the Iron Dome had just started protecting the country with about fifty percent success. They had sent for Max to eliminate a particular Hamas leader in southern Lebanon who had orchestrated the rocket launches from Gaza. Nowadays, things were calmer, so Max couldn't guess what was so urgent that Rosh would summon him back. Eventually, he felt himself slipping off to sleep. Any further interpretation would have to wait.

The next morning, Max and Lilah awoke and spent their unannounced day off catching up. They walked along the beach and had coffee and croissants at their favorite beach café. Later in the morning, Lilah visited her parents' home next door to Max's Aunt Gila. Max got a ride to see his friends at RAMOW.

CHAPTER 30

Hidden in plain sight in the middle of a thick grove of orange trees was a shrub-obscured entrance. The driver had left Max off nearby, where he pulled his carry-on through a doorway. An electric steel door closed behind him. After negotiating two different levels of military security, Max had entered the three-story underground fortress and found himself in an enormous elevator, big enough to hold a pick-up truck. It carried Max down ten meters below the ground level to a spacious center room. He greeted the few members of the team at their desks with a warm "Shalom."

RAMOW, an acronym for the Rafael-Mossad Center for Offensive Strategic Development and Weisman Institute, was the R & D division of the Mossad. With a four-meter ceiling, the large central core contained curved desks scattered around the circular room. Multiple desktop computers with large screens stood like trees on work surfaces. Some were vertically oriented as needed with CAD/CAM software. Others had Apple Mac Pro computers with large double studio screens.

A round counter height table stood in the center of the space, surrounded by twelve high stools for the team members. Four doors located around the room's circumference connected the central core to different workrooms. Each workroom provided other functions, including engineering, biological science, weaponry, and mechanics.

The space was impenetrable by any modern-day electronics or conventional weapons. The kibbutzniks who picked the oranges each summer had no idea of the novel inventions and top-secret decisions being made below them. None of the RAMOW team lived on the kibbutz; they just worked there.

Despite having no natural sunlight, the rooms were well lit, bright, and cheerful. Soft pastel-colored fabric covered the contemporary office furniture. The largest wall surrounded 50% of the circular room and functioned as a giant white erase board. The smooth white surface displayed various handwritten formulas, calculations, and outlines. RAMOW's team members did their math and other challenging calculations in full view of the team, which encouraged collaboration.

The people who worked there were compulsively organized and felt like a family. As Max approached the team members, he was greeted with a warm embrace from the beautiful Bina.

"It makes it worth the whole trip just to be hugged by you," said Max.

"Oh, you say that to all the women," Bina responded, laughing, and rolling her eyes.

"Not really. No woman I know embraces me like you do."

"How about Lilah?" said Bina with a wink.

He looked down, hiding his smile, and didn't have a retort. "Lilah was a fortunate woman," continued Bina. "I'd love to meet her someday."

"Maybe you will," said Max.

"Lilah is lucky I'm a lesbian," Bina laughed.

Gaining his composure which he rarely lost, "Bina," he declared, admiring her attractive five-foot-ten-inch frame, "you are too much! Someday, you'll meet Lilah, and until then, you and the work of the RAMOW team will remain a secret from her and the rest of the world!"

As they were chatting, Lev approached and greeted Max with the usual bro-hug. "Welcome, Max," he said. "How did things go in Colorado?"

"Your equipment performed perfectly. Thank you," said Max. "My problem is that someone figured out that it was not an accident. Worse, three days later, a hit team came to our Boston condo to kill me."

Lev's eyes widened in shock, "Oh my gosh, Max. Is there anything we can do to help?"

"There are a few things, probably unrelated." Max opened the carry-on he was pulling. "In one night, six men died in a St. Thomas hotel. One of those victims was my cardiac team nurse. That's how I got involved. In each of these reinforced sealed plastic bags is a motion-sensitive air freshener I pilfered from the hotel. One is heavier than the other. I have no idea if they are related to the deaths, but I was curious what you might find. Please take absolute HAZMAT precautions."

Lev texted Ivan to join them. When Ivan entered, Lev said, "Hey MacIvan, Max has something for you."

Ivan hugged Max and said, "It's great to see you. What's up?"

Max explained the story to Ivan. "I'll let you know what we find," said Ivan, as he carefully took the bags and left the room.

Lev and Max spoke for a while before Max left for a ride to headquarters in the outskirts of Tel Aviv. After the hidden turn-off Altneuland Road, the driver dropped him off just past the entrance to the Gliliot Military Base.

Out front of the nondescript concrete building, Max approached and smiled at the two quite serious guards on either side of the entrance. Although the guards recognized him, he still had to place both hands on the large pads on the countertop and look straight into the camera for the combination of facial and handprint recognition. Then, he took the elevator up to the top floor of the austere building. The concrete walls were half a meter thick, and the small glass windows were bulletproof. The windows were too small for a person to fit through, but there were well-placed, hidden escape chutes out the sides of the building.

He made his way to the anteroom of the Director's office. Max knocked loudly on the door. Before he could say anything, he heard Ahuvi yell, "Get in here, Maxy!"

"*Shalom*, Madame Executive Assistant. How did you know it was me?"

"No one knocks like you do, Max. Most are afraid to knock with more than a little tap. Like the door will break or something." Ahuvi gave Max a smirk. "These guys are supposed to be killers, but they can't even knock!" in the same breath, "Where have you been?" She asked this with a smile, knowing full well that he had left Boston two days before and had spent time with Lilah.

Disregarding her question, as Max often did, he protested, "Oh, Ahuvi, don't look at me like that!" He returned her smile. "Will the boss be off his phone soon?"

She looked up quickly in astonishment. "How did you know he was on the phone?"

Max had noticed the lit button of the Director's extension on her desk phone. He said, "Well, you always say he is on the phone when I call."

Although her actual title was executive assistant, Ahuvi was the commander-in-chief of this space in front of the Director's office. She knew every agent by name and things about them that didn't appear in their personnel files. The current Mossad director was the third she'd supported. The Director didn't give her orders; his directives were more like suggestions or requests. Fortunately for Max, he was her favorite agent.

The Director's door opened, and before he could say anything, Max spoke: "It's so good to see you. I hope you didn't miss me."

"Shut up and get in here," said Rosh irritably as he led Max into the office.

"*Shalom* to you as well," Max said, winking at Ahuvi. He had barely gotten into the office before Rosh slammed the door behind him.

CHAPTER 31

As soon as the Group's Chairman finished thanking Brandt, Amir—who had been silent throughout the meeting—suddenly blurted out, "Dr. Brandt, I am fascinated by what your clinical trials have shown and by your proposal. If you desire educated and experienced personnel, I can supply them." He was already thinking about how he could provide a larger space and the financing for Jaeger's research, without the Group's involvement. But he kept that to himself. "We share the same goal," he said simply.

"Yes, of course, Mr. Khan," Jaeger answered reluctantly. He tried to hide his discomfort at the thought of working with an Arab.

"The Group would like to see the two of you move forward on this project together," the Chairman cut in.

"Yes, sir," said Jaeger, wondering how this was going to work. Staring straight at Amir, he said, "Whatever you wish." He didn't sense any compatibility with Mr. Khan, and he preferred to work alone. But Brandt needed the Group's support and thus would abide by their rules. He had to admit that the Arab filled him with some curiosity. Could Khan deliver on what he said?

At the end of the meeting, Jaeger turned to Amir, testing the extent of his commitment, "Mr. Khan, I will need more laboratory space and trained technicians, men experienced working in laboratories, listening to orders, and trusted. Can you have your men available for me by next week?"

"Yes, the additional technicians you need will be available next week. As a start, I was thinking of sending you four experienced microbiology researchers—women, actually— to help you grow the virus. When you are ready for more assistants, you'll let me know. And you said you need more space. Would you permit me to see your laboratory so I can get a sense of what you need?"

"I have not had to work with women laboratory assistants since my fellowship days," Dr. Brandt said with disdain. "They were more of a distraction than a help. Do you think *your* women can be helpful and take instruction?"

Amir realized he was dealing with a troublesome man. He assured Jaeger that if the women proved useless, he would replace them with men after a week.

Before Jaeger could respond, Gustav interjected, "Good. The two of you can work out the logistics later. The Khan family has smuggled people and armaments in and out of Europe and the US for years. I am sure you two will resolve any challenges and deliver an effective product as we approach our goals. Any further questions?" The way the Chairman asked, he was not inviting a response.

The meeting ended abruptly. The duo who had welcomed Jaeger and Amir now escorted the two visitors out. Walking to the elevator, Amir turned to Jaeger, holding out his hand. About to withdraw, Jaeger, with a tight face, was slow to lift his hand to meet Amir's.

"It was a privilege to meet you, Dr. Brandt."

Jaeger wasn't so sure. He didn't trust Amir. The man was articulate, well dressed, and poised, a walking contradiction of Jaeger's stereotypes about Arabs. *And now he wants to visit my laboratory*, Jaeger thought. No outsiders see my laboratory!

Jaeger met Amir's intensely dark eyes above a partial smile in a poker face. The scientist didn't like that he couldn't tell what Amir was thinking.

Was the man's charm genuine? He felt the Arab's firm, cool handshake while hoping his own soft, moist hand wasn't sweating excessively.

"I admire what you have accomplished in your research," Amir said. He could sense that this weird, cold, awkward professor type was uncomfortable with him, so he turned on his sycophantic persona. "Doctor, we have much more in common than you can imagine. In short, we have the same enemies. And the enemy of my enemy is my friend. So, please allow me to buy you a drink back at the hotel. I have a proposal that I know you will embrace."

After their guests left the meeting, the Group of four looked at each other. Gustav Schröder, an Austrian businessman and founder of the Group, spoke first. "What do you think?"

"I don't know if the two of them can even sit in the same room again," said Altman Ansel, a German industrialist. "Brandt looked like he was going to faint when you suggested they should collaborate."

"I don't like Khan," said Domenico Bernard, a Swiss banker. "He'd sooner slit Brandt's throat than work with him."

"He'd probably slit all our throats if the circumstances were right," said Beau Lancelot, the French High-Tech Entrepreneur.

"I hope all of you are wrong," said Gustav cheerfully. "Let's see what this unlikely duo can accomplish. They may surprise us."

CHAPTER 32

The same driver who had brought Dr. Brandt to the meeting was waiting outside the building and drove Jaeger and Amir back to the refurbished classic pre-war hotel. The two men didn't speak a word in the car, until the driver dropped them off. Walking into the hotel, they agreed to meet in the bar in thirty minutes.

Amir's cell phone buzzed on his way to his hotel room, and he looked at the screen. There were five messages, all from the same number that he didn't recognize. *International,* he thought. *A U.S. number?* He called the number back.

"*As-salamu-alaykum,* sir, this is Mohammad."

Amir responded, "*Wa'alaykumu s-salam.* Nice to hear your voice again, Mohammad. Are you still in Boston?"

"Sir, I am calling from Sommerville, Massachusetts, just outside Boston. We received communication about the man who murdered your brother. A few days ago, we sent two men to kill him."

Interrupting, Amir said, "That's wonderful."

"Well, sir, apparently they failed," Mohammad said cautiously.

"I don't understand. What happened?" asked Amir, incredulous.

"Sir, our two men disappeared. They visited the building where the target lived. It took two days for us to learn that the building's concierge was shot and taken to a hospital. He is still alive. As I mentioned, we have lost our brethren, and we have no way of knowing what happened."

"Tell me the name of the murderer," Amir demanded.

"We have it on good authority that his name is Max Dent, and he is a surgeon living in Boston," said Mohammad. "I will text you a photo we found on the Internet."

Overwhelmed with the thought that he now knew the identity of his brother's murderer, Amir could scarcely control himself. Trying to calm himself down, he said, "Failure is unacceptable. Find the man and kill him." Then Amir ended the phone call and sat down on his bed to gather his thoughts before going downstairs to meet Brandt.

It was late in the evening, but the hotel bar was not quieting down. The music was loud enough that even people sitting together could hardly hear each other. About fifteen visitors sat on cushioned stools around the bar.

When Jaeger arrived, precisely thirty minutes after the driver had dropped them off, Amir was already at a high-top table with an open bottle of champagne and two glasses. Despite his Muslim faith, business was business, and a drink was an excellent way to start a new venture.

He lifted his full glass of champagne towards Jaeger and toasted: "To success in our joint mission."

Jaeger reluctantly lifted the filled glass of chilled champagne, thinking that this was one thing the French did well. He tapped Amir's glass with his own and drank it down. He held his glass out for barely two seconds before Amir refilled it. As Brandt sipped it, he felt a buzz coming on.

Jaeger whispered the second toast, "To the Group!" After several more toasts, Jaeger softened. Amir ordered a second bottle.

"Sir, I feel you're getting me drunk," slurred Jaeger.

Wanting to take full advantage of Jaeger's need for self-importance, Amir continued, "Please, Dr. Brandt! We are only celebrating your incredible scientific achievements. You deserve a larger party, but that's not possible now as your brilliant discoveries must remain our secret."

Jaeger noted the "we" and the "our" in Amir's words. Jaeger now had a partner, whether he liked it or not.

Amir continued, "It amazes me you can selectively kill cells in a human just by releasing some vapor. The implications for modern medicine are astounding. I assume you plan to use your new technology for curing cancers."

Brandt forced a laugh. "The biggest cancer I wish to rid the world of is the Jews." He punched the palm of his other hand for emphasis. "The problem is, just like there are many cancers, there are many types of Jews. So, I have been trying to find genetic blends that will selectively kill as large a Jewish population as possible. But," Jaeger gulped down a glass of water, realizing Amir would never understand the science, "let's just say that Jews vary like the rest of the world. There are many genetic variations among them."

Amir had always thought a Jew was a Jew, but Jaeger described in more detail than Amir could comprehend the different types of Jews he could kill and why doing so would require multiple modifications of the lethal virus. Jaeger explained at length how he had been working on Ashkenazi and Sephardic genetic identities.

"Someday, with a big enough laboratory and my technology," he said proudly, "I'll be able to identify the genetic code of every human being. And once I have that inventory—" he raised his glass to toast again, although Amir's glass had remained empty for some time— "nothing can stop me!"

"That's unbelievable," said Amir. "How much of this have you shared with the Group?"

"They don't know of the challenges. They don't want to hear about the problems, just the solutions."

"What sort of problems?" Despite his strong desire to work with Brandt, Amir worried that this all might be a sham. "Is there something I can do to help you resolve the problems?" asked Amir.

Trying to figure out how to answer without appearing desperate, Jaeger said, "More manpower is all I need," said Jaeger. "More help and a bigger lab."

"Well then," Amir leaned forward, with his elbows on the table, "I can arrange that. How else can I help you with your clinical trials? If you are considering new targets, why don't we start by killing Jews in Israel? My Palestinian brothers would love to strike back at the occupying infidels. I am ready to deploy your virus when you are ready to trust me."

As he felt Amir's face coming closer to his own, Jaeger's suspicions rose. He was feeling tipsy and having a hard time holding a thought in his head. Finally pointing his accusing finger at Amir, he said, "You are pushing me."

"Not at all. You said you needed more assistants and more space. Would you be willing to show me your laboratory so I can get a sense of what you need?"

Jaeger froze. He was not sure about bringing this stranger into his lab. "Why do you want to see my lab?" he said suspiciously. "It's just a typical research laboratory."

Amir kept his cool and persisted. "Based on the scientific discoveries you shared with the Group, I have a feeling it is not just a typical lab. You are doing world-class work! And I want to help you grow your success. But, Dr. Brandt, we need to trust each other if we collaborate as the Group has requested. The reason I want to see your lab is that I'd like to get a sense of how many assistants you have room for at present."

Jaeger was still skeptical. To trust anyone enough to partner with him—let alone this Arab—was a tall order. "I am flying home tomorrow morning and returning to my lab from the airport. Let me think about it, and let's continue this conversation tomorrow." And with that, Jaeger said good night and went to his room for a much-needed sleep.

Amir realized he might have been pushing the German too hard, but he had to make this happen. After paying the check, he went to his room, and packed his bag, and checked out of the hotel. There were things to arrange. The pilots were told to meet him at the Nuremberg airport and have the plane ready in one hour for a trip to Rostock-Laage Airport. Sleeping on his aircraft was far more comfortable and safer than the hotel.

As he boarded the private jet, Amir's mind was practically exploding with ideas. He was incredulous that this German scientist had the power of the gods in his hands. Amir had to figure out how to use this weapon for its broadest effect. He could see it all now: beginning in Israel, the PLO and Hamas would push out the remaining Jews, making a seismic change in the Middle East and the world. Israel would fall to its knees to stop the deaths of nearly all its Jews. He could then focus his budget on terrorism in the west. *It is Allah's will,* Amir told himself.

Amir's responsibility to the Prince obliged him to give the monarch an update before launching into the next phase of the planning. In their last meeting, before Amir had left for Germany, the Prince had granted Amir full access to one of the royal family's jets for the month—if he stayed within Europe and avoided France and the Middle East. Since the fiasco in Colorado, no more trips to the U.S., either. France was out because they boycotted Saudi oil.

In addition to offering his jet, the Prince had put up five million euros to support the infrastructure of the Khan family's terrorist plan, along with another three million euros for any unanticipated expenses, such as in Germany. Some of the money would be used to support the growth of Brandt's lab. The Prince wouldn't want to know any details. Still, Amir knew the Prince would be much happier supporting terrorist activities than trying to fight a war the old-fashioned way, beholden to the incompetent Saudi military.

As he listened to the dial tone, waiting for the Prince to answer from the royal family's palace in Riyadh, Amir felt happier than he had since before his brother's death.

CHAPTER 33

At Mossad headquarters, Rosh stared at Max, who now sat calmly across the desk from him. Rosh was incredulous that it had taken him an extra day to show up in his office. "Your lack of gratitude is remarkable," Rosh stated loudly. "I extended myself immediately to get you and your girlfriend out of a dangerous situation, and you put me off till now?"

The new Director of the Mossad was the first in the history of the Israeli intelligence service not to have been an experienced spy before ascending to the post. Although everyone called him Rosh, his actual name was Shmuel Gurion. Everyone at the Mossad knew he had gotten the job as a political appointment—or political compromise. The grandson of Israel's first prime minister, Shmuel, was a brilliant mathematician who had studied at the Technion, Oxford, and then Stanford before returning to Israel to start a highly successful telecom company. The fortune he'd made by the young age of thirty-five had allowed him to donate large amounts of money to certain political campaigns in Israel.

Shmuel had always been a smooth operator. He'd befriended the politicians who shared his philosophy of making strategic investments in futuristic military technology and who had invited him to chair the new High-Tech Intelligence Committee for the Knesset, Israel's parliament.

Once Shmuel's friend of twenty years became Prime Minister, Shmuel got the chance to lead the Mossad. Rosh, as he was now called, knew more than anyone about the technology and communications the agents used, but he knew nothing about killing people. He hadn't shot a gun since his service in the IDF over forty years ago.

Max interrupted, "We're very grateful to you, sir. But you know, family first! So now, I'm here at your service." Max hated kowtowing to this underqualified bully, but he knew he had to stay in line to manage him effectively.

"How much did you share with Lilah?" asked Rosh.

"Everything," said Max in a neutral tone.

With a remarkably unanimated face staring into Max's eyes, Rosh demanded, "What the hell were you doing in St. Thomas? What was so important—vacation?" Before Max could answer, the Director waved his hand dismissively. "I don't care. We have more important things to discuss."

Rosh launched into his tale. "I got a call from the CIA Director, Cummings, a few days ago. He began by asking if we remembered the bombing attack in Jerusalem three years ago that killed a group of Israeli and Palestinian teenage soccer players. I told him we remember every bombing that happens in our country." He jabbed his finger on the desk angrily and continued, "We'll never forget: the kids were playing on the same team together, and this asshole terrorist kills them all. The Palestinian community blamed the Israelis, and the Israeli community did the opposite. How could we not remember?"

"For obvious reasons, the CIA got excited because they see a connection between that event and the recent death of a Saudi skier in Aspen. An astute FBI agent in Denver, Walid Manzur—who happens to be a Lebanese-American Muslim—believed the skier was not killed by accident. This agent paid a visit to Dani, the *sayan* hairstylist. Fortunately, Manzur was too late to recover your things." Max did his best not to betray any anxiety as Rosh recited these facts. "So, I ask myself, are they fishing —" he shot Max an intense look— "or do they know?"

"There is no way they can connect the dead skier with us or with me," Max said confidently. "Everything went as planned. They have no weapon and no witness."

"Well, my dear Max, for once, you are wrong. The FBI guessed that the skier would have tried to avoid the tree he hit, but his tracks suggested otherwise. They have a photograph of the dead skier, and it shows his ski tracks. Their report said the skier lost control before he hit the tree."

Max let out a sigh. "The damn ski tracks," he muttered, more to himself than to Rosh. "I can't believe I missed that." He met Rosh's gaze. "They *were* fishing. They may have gotten lucky, but they were fishing," said Max, inwardly cursing his oversight.

Rosh smiled inside, knowing that he had just cut the famous Max Dent down to size. And now he had Max where he needed him.

"Max, I don't care about the fucking CIA. We have a bigger problem, and I need your help. Something has been brewing in Europe. We have few details. Someone has hoarded tons of cash in a small bank in Switzerland. Over the last two years the Wulff AG Zurich bank has accumulated over 100 million euros in one account."

"A Swiss bank receiving a sizeable amount of money? Doesn't seem unusual," said Max with a slight smirk, but he contained his sarcasm. He knew Rosh was trapping him into a new mission.

Rosh ignored him. "The sources of the money were an unusual mix. Initially, the money originated from three countries: Germany, France, Austria. In the last three months, people in America and Saudi Arabia have joined in. In each of the countries, the money originated in one bank before being wired to Wulff. So far, we identified one donor, a third-generation industrialist and machine manufacturer whose family thrived off the Germano-Austrian war industry of the 1930s. He identifies as an Austrian, and his company manufactured parts required for the engines in all German cars, trucks, and trains. He also made parts for virtually every sports car engine in the world."

"Four years ago, his company had never transferred a penny to any Swiss bank. In the last two years, there has been a steady flow of euros to one account at Wulff AG Zurich. He used a dummy corporate account in Bermuda, where we picked up the money trail. The money arrived gradually, via circuitous routes, for deposit in the Swiss bank. And the thing is, after tracking this process for several years, we haven't been able to identify any investment opportunity or purpose for this secret, laundered money. We know that the guy had been a major donor to extreme right-wing, anti-Semitic political campaigns in the past."

"It sounds suspicious, sir, but accusing the Swiss of harboring dirty money in their banks is like asking the Orthodox to untie the knots on their *tzitzis*. It's unthinkable. So why are you telling me this story?"

Ignoring Max's comment again, the Director went on. "If the money is being stashed to finance terrorism, it's enough for a lot of attacks, or maybe one big one," Rosh noted. "Cash has only been coming in so far, not going out. That is the problem. If the money is being dispersed, we couldn't find it."

"Rosh, this all sounds fascinating—but again, why are you speaking with me about it? We had an agreement: the Colorado assignment was a one-off. And, given that it didn't go as desired, I don't know why you still want—."

Cutting Max off, Rosh continued, "We have to find everyone involved in this scheme. A bunch of people has stockpiled all this money, and it seems they want to change the course of European history! I told you, the Austrian donor is a known anti-Semite. For all we know, their plan may involve killing Jews and probably eradicating Israel while they're at it. So Max," he said, leaning forward on his desk and looking Max in the eye at last, "the threat is real."

Curious but not giving in, Max asked, "Is there any evidence that these depositors are financing terrorism?" He gave Rosh a stern look. "I figured you must have had something to justify springing for the private jet to get Lilah and me back to Israel," he said at last.

"I flew you home immediately because your lives were in danger, and you weren't free to act in the U.S. Also, yes, I needed you here to help solve this problem. Listen, I know we don't always…I mean, whatever. What I am trying to say is, you're the best we have, and with RAMOW's help, I pray you can solve this riddle and expose these assholes in Europe. I am convinced they want to do us harm."

Max didn't respond directly but asked, "Rosh, how did the Saudis get to me so quickly? They came to my home. They could have hurt Lilah. Let's talk about that."

"I don't know, Max, and I'm sorry. If it came from the family of the guy you knocked off, well, that would be a surprise. We thought when we cut off the head, the snake would die." Rosh's expression was grim. "This snake may have another head."

"Tell me what I don't know about the Kahn family," Max demanded.

Rosh hoped the direction of this conversation would get Max to cooperate. He said with conviction, "His father is senile. Asif's siblings were twins, a boy, and a girl. As far as we know, neither involved themselves in terrorist activities. The sister's a physician-scientist who did research at a lab in Riyadh. We have photos of her and their brother. We know little about the brother. He was educated in the United States, I think at Harvard. But the older brother, Asif, the one you killed, did all the dirty work. The bomber for that soccer match in Jerusalem three years ago got his bomb from Asif Khan. Directly or indirectly, he has been responsible for many focused attacks, including the legendary one in Spain."

"Yeah," said Max, "But how did they find me in Boston?"

"Anyway, our agents in Boston," Rosh continued, "verified that the guys who came to your condo were Wahhabi followers."

"Doubt that we've heard the last from that family or their followers. Maybe someone else was calling the shots." Max speculated.

"I don't know, but we'll try to find out. It's probably coming from the Kingdom. Look, Max, I am concerned about your safety. But I'm *very* concerned about the money transfers in Europe. I don't trust anybody with that many hidden assets. If right-wing Austrians and Germans are behind this, it can't be good for Israel. And what are they doing collaborating with the Saudis? That much money could buy a lot of terrorist munitions and reimbursements for the families of suicide bombers. We must find out what their plan is. I have already spoken with the Prime Minister. He has given this project top priority and his blessing."

Max had grown quiet. Rosh had built a good case, and Max could see he was stuck in the middle of it. He wished he'd never taken on the Colorado assignment.

Rosh's voice broke in again. "Max, you probably figured out what we're thinking: that the family of the schmuck you killed in Aspen might be behind the influx of Saudi cash into those bank accounts. He was also, most likely, the financier who paid for the suicide vests and bombs those two terrorists used when they killed your family twenty-five years ago. Of all people, I don't need to tell you, that in Gaza and the West Bank, hundreds of young fanatics are training to be martyrs for future attacks. This dirty money keeps it going."

"So," Max spoke at last, "If there's a connection between the hoarded European money and the Wahabbi terrorist network—"

Rosh finished his sentence, "The problems are bigger than we feared. For all we know, they may have a WMD that they could deliver to our doorstep. One of our *sayans* reported that Asif Khan had made a trip to Europe three months before his last trip to Colorado. When our enemies unite, our challenges grow exponentially."

Max stared at Rosh for a moment, then closed his eyes. He had come to Israel seeking refuge from the threats on U.S. soil. Assuming his Mossad activities were done, Max had told Lilah everything. But now, he thought wearily, it seemed like he was right back in it. Worse—he was in deeper than ever! What would Lilah say?

Rosh barreled on: "Your little activity in Colorado grew wings. Our friends in the CIA were very disappointed that we acted on their soil without getting permission from them and the FBI. Fuck that! We denied any relationship and told them they are just pulling at straws. But Max, they identified you as being a skier on the mountain. Ironically, they used the latest Israeli recognition software to find you! We told them you were there coincidentally, as a heart surgeon attending a medical conference in Aspen. Just an unfortunate coincidence, we told them."

Max grimaced. "I don't know, sir. Killing a high-profile Saudi terrorist on American soil may not have been our cleverest idea. On the other hand, the FBI is ruthless in solving murders. What additional information did your CIA contact tell you?" asked Max.

"Apparently, that Denver FBI agent suspected foul play. Right now, they don't trust that the CIA told them everything." Tightening his lips and tapping his fingers on the desk, his tension mounting, Rosh admitted, "And they'd be correct in that assumption."

Max felt incredibly tired. "How did the Arabs identify me?"

"I don't know."

"I should have brushed away the tracks!" Max shook his head, frustrated with himself. "I had to get away before another skier saw me. It was a plan with too much risk. *What was I thinking?*"

"We can assume the FBI worked on the photo and verified the victim's identity. That's how the CIA found out, and they are now furious with me for not including them in the plan. I guarantee we haven't heard the end of this," finished Rosh.

Max suddenly felt that he didn't want to continue this conversation. He needed time to think. "Sir, I need to go; I'm sorry," he snapped. "I'll be in touch." And with that, Max got up and walked out.

Rosh looked up from his seated position. "What do you mean, you're leaving? You can't just walk out of my office like that!" He was still yelling at Max's back as the door closed.

CHAPTER 34

The driver Ahuvi had arranged was waiting when Max got outside. Before getting in the car, he called Aunt Gila that he was on his way. He'd tried to tell Rosh he wouldn't continue to work for the Mossad. But, having learned about the alleged conspiracy beginning in Europe, how could he stick to his demands? His phone ringing interrupted his thoughts.

"Max, I have been trying to reach you," said Dr. Anthony Dibona. "We completed the autopsy on your nurse, David Springs. As you suspected, he died from a severe respiratory illness. He had hemorrhagic sputum and mucus and hemorrhagic congestion in the lungs and bronchi. The alveoli in the lungs were full of the same bloody mucus you saw in the nostrils. This was a diffuse destructive pneumonia from a severe viral respiratory infection, maybe influenza. But I know that sounds crazy."

"Why is it so crazy?" asked Max.

"There is no flu epidemic in St Thomas or anywhere else in the world right now. Max, what's going on there?"

"I don't know and share your concern. Thank you, Tony, for doing the autopsy."

"Of course. I notified the deceased's family, and the funeral home has already picked up the body. The funeral is tomorrow. I had the hospital cover all the additional costs."

"Thank you for that as well," said Max. "And Tony, I have another question. When I was at the morgue in St. Thomas, there were five other bodies that came in the same day from the same hotel, and one more guy was dying in the ICU from respiratory failure. All had the same bloody mucus-stained clothes and bloody discharge from their nostrils that David's body and clothes revealed."

"Oh my gosh," said Tony, whose voice's pitch had raised an octave. "It sounds like a contagion…but no one else in the hotel got sick, right?"

"That's correct, as far as I know," answered Max.

Tony spoke more slowly, "Since this may be a contagious infection, I have to report our case to the Department of Public Health. Just letting you know. Also, I'll reach out to the pathologist at the St. Thomas Hospital. Hopefully he'll discuss the case with me, and we can share our findings. It's awful, but now I'm intrigued."

"That would be great," said Max. "Let me know if you find anything else."

Max got in the car. With traffic, the fifteen-minute ride would take longer, giving Max time to strategize. The driver took him the fourteen kilometers northeast to Ra'anana. Max smiled as he approached his neighborhood, feeling a deep warm sensation returning home. His memories of those eleven years calling Gila's place home were mixed. This was the town where he had become a man and had buried his family. He had developed his warrior skills in the IDF and the Sayeret Matkal. Seeing the street sign of their road: Meraglim Street, made him smile. The Biblical Meraglim were the twelve spies sent out by Moses to scout the land that would become Israel. Maybe it was prophetic.

The small stucco home, with three bedrooms on two floors, sat five meters from identical dwellings on either side. One belonged to Lilah's parents, an older German-born couple who, as children, had survived the

Holocaust by escaping to Israel. Late in their lives, they had finally conceived one child, a daughter. Aunt Gila stood on the front steps to welcome Max.

Hugging him with a full-body squeeze, Gila exclaimed with tears in her eyes, "Max, baby, you are even more handsome than when I saw you last!"

"Aunt Gila, you look more beautiful than ever," he answered as they embraced with warm cheek-to-cheek kisses. He was nearly a foot taller, yet he felt safe and comforted in her presence. Gila bore a strong resemblance to his father, her older brother— not in size, but in character. She shared her late brother's sense of fairness and modesty; also, as a formidable, vocal advocate for Israel.

"You know Max, I miss our time together."

With his hands on her shoulders, looking down at her smiling face, "I miss our moments, too," responded Max, "our walks."

"You used to ask me so many questions," said Gila. "I couldn't believe how wise you were at such a young age. You kept me on my toes."

Max smiled. "Aunt Gila, you were my world."

"Also, you had such rage," Gila said in an understanding tone. "We spent a lot of time just talking about revenge. Do you remember that?" asked Gila.

"Yes, I do. And I recall your quoting from Confucius: 'A man who acts to seek revenge should dig two graves, one for himself.'" Getting more serious for a moment, he said, "That's truer than I realized at the time."

Picking up on his change in tone, she asked, "What do you mean?"

Changing the subject, Max said, "Gila, it's great to see you. I can smell my favorite brisket in the oven!"

"Bullshit!" Gila laughed. "If you missed me so much, you would have visited sooner!" Animating the phrases with her hands, as she often did, she emphasized every word. "You never write, and you're not on Facebook. When they write about you on your hospital's website, that's where I learn you are still alive!" she said with a smile. "Why didn't you bring our beautiful Lilah with you?" asked Gila. "The Fischers would have loved to see her."

"We flew home together. She is probably out with her parents now. I'm sure she could use a day off from me to process things…" Max trailed off.

"Process what things?" Gila picked up on this right away.

After a moment, he answered, "Until last night, Lilah didn't know the extent of my work as a *kidon* in the Mossad."

Gila, who fussed around her kitchen to get Max a cup of tea, stopped in her tracks and looked at him. "What do you mean, she didn't know?"

"It's complicated."

She shook her head, forming a prayer position with her hands, palms touching in front of her lips, as she always did when making a point, "My guess is, she knew, but she didn't *acknowledge*. She was always a smart girl and had a sixth sense about things—just like you. I sometimes describe it to my friends with that line from the Star Wars movie: you have the 'Force.' You both do."

Max chuckled, "Gila, let's not get carried away."

"It's true, Max! Lilah has a similar skill. It's a good thing for a psychiatrist to have a sense about their patients and a heightened awareness of things around her." As she bustled around the kitchen, Gila went on, "Max, I've got a story you may not have heard. When she was a young teenager, maybe fourteen, she came home and noticed two Arab strangers loitering further down Meraglim from our home. Without being noticed, she slowly turned around, walked in the other direction, and knocked on the door of a neighbor. She used their phone to summon the police. The police surrounded the neighborhood. Thanks to Lilah, the police disarmed the strangers before they could trigger suicide vests. Lilah probably saved my life and the lives of her family and the neighbors. She thinks on her feet and is fearless—like you."

Gila turned off the stove; the kettle had boiled. She poured Max a cup of tea. "And besides," she said, gesturing with her arms outspread, "everyone I know thinks that you were Mossad."

Max was still thinking about what Gila had just told him. "Lilah never told me that story." But he thought to himself, there were probably more she didn't share. He continued, "I guess each of us has been keeping secrets."

Max helped Gila clear the plates after enjoying his favorite home-cooked meal. At last, he said, "The Mossad wants me active. They have more work for me to do."

"Is that what *you* want?" Gila asked, meeting his gaze.

Max shook his head, "I am committed to being a heart surgeon in Boston. I don't want the double life anymore."

Gila kept staring into his eyes for a moment and then said, "Let's take a walk." They went outside. The sun was low approaching the horizon, and a gentle spring breeze cooled the air. The street was quiet. Gila held his hand as they walked. Since he was thirteen, the two of them had walked together holding hands.

Max knew this was Gila's preferred setting for their serious talks. Squeezing his hand as she often did for emphasis, glimpsing his blue eyes in the darkened street, Gila began, "Max, first and always, you are a Jew and an Israeli. I know you care for many people. But no one except Jews looks out for Jews. I admire the work you do to fix patients' hearts. But who will protect Israel's heart?"

Max stared at the tall, majestic eucalyptus trees that lined Meraglim street. The leaves were just filling out and growing grand shadows. He realized these trees had witnessed his transformation into a man and Israel's evolution into a modern world power. She went on. "You are a *sabra*. This land is your land. No one else understands the meaning of *Eretz Israel* as you do. Who better to protect it? Do you know something, Max? Many people, including myself, sleep better because of what people like you do. You are out there making us safe. I love you so much, I worry for your safety. But I would never discourage you from fighting the lifelong battle for Israel."

Silence ensued before Max spoke. "You always have a way of clarifying my confusion. Sometimes I feel like two people in one life, and each battling for primacy. I feel pressure to choose one path." He paused and looked at Gila earnestly, but he could sense the tiredness in his expression. "Do you think I will ever be able to leave the Mossad?"

"I think you have dedicated your life to protecting and healing others. To preventing harm. You're in this now, and I think your conscience won't rest until you've seen it through to a natural conclusion."

They stood quietly on the sidewalk, a few blocks down from Gila's home. Max was thinking about how to manage his relationship with Lilah. Could she be in his life without risking her own? If he continued his Mossad activities, could they continue to live safely in Boston? Of course, living in Israel would be safer—but what about his surgical practice?

"There's still enough light out; let's go for a ride," Gila said suddenly. "I'm driving!"

She drove her blue Mazda with abandon till they arrived at the Kiryat Shaul Cemetery in northern Tel Aviv. It was early evening. The sun was continuing down casting long shadows beneath the trees. Gila parked in her usual spot. They walked in silence, hand in hand, towards the family plot. Max recalled how Aunt Gila had taken him by the hand many times over the years to walk to the graves of his parents, his mother's and father's parents, his brother Bruce, and Gila's husband, Samuel. Gila pointed out how the trees' soft shadows lined up like mourners at a funeral. Max saw them as soldiers guarding the sacred ground.

They stared at the graves. Finally, after a few minutes of silence, Max spoke: "There is something very calming about being here." Tears started down his cheeks. He could not help but relive the explosion and seeing his family strewn around the room. The sense of helplessness tightened his gut as he recalled getting out from under the table. He could not forgive himself for surviving.

After a few more minutes of silence, looking up at Max's teary face, Gila spoke, "Max, that feeling burns in all our souls. As Jews, we just want to live our lives. We just want to be left alone to be free and live safely. But for as long as two people want to claim the same land, each will lay claim at the expense of the other. We either fight for and defend our land or be destroyed by the other. Your home is here. It has always been. That's why you will always find your way back."

"We never brought Lilah here," Max said suddenly. "She was too young when our family was killed. I really didn't know her until she got to Boston," said Max.

Gila shook her head. "That's not exactly accurate." Gila squeezed Max's hand more tightly. "During one of Lilah's trips home from Boston, I think before she had moved in with you, she visited me. She told me she'd met you in Boston and that she was falling in love with you. We spoke for a while; then I drove her here. I wanted her to hear the story from me. She cried that day, the way you just did. You know, Lilah loves Israel as you do. It's in her blood."

The two remaining Dent family members focused on the cemetery markers covered with little stones for a while longer. Then, as the sun went below the horizon, they hugged and left.

Once they were back at Aunt Gila's home, Max took a cab to the condo in Natanya for the night. He got a text from Lilah that made him smile. She would be spending the evening at her parents' home in Ra'anana.

Max felt overwhelmed by the day's events. First things first, he told himself. It was seven hours earlier in Boston, but it was Saturday. He emailed his executive assistant that he would be away for a month to deal with a family issue. Knowing all the scheduled patients by name, he helped his assistant prioritize referrals to his colleagues. As usual, Gila was right. There was more he had to do. The only way out was through.

CHAPTER 35

The following day, a cold, overcast sky threatened snow over the Rostock-Laage Airport. Despite the gloomy weather, Amir felt rested, wearing a fresh shirt and a neatly pressed suit.

Jaeger landed and climbed down the stairs. Standing on the Tarmac, Amir surprised him. His presence unnerved Brandt, making his hands sweat.

As Amir thrust his hand forward to shake, Brandt stood still and kept his hands on the two bags he was carrying.

"Dr. Brandt, I am sorry to startle you. How was your flight?"

"Fine," Jaeger snapped. "What are you doing here?"

Amir lied, "I just flew in a little before you. May I assume you are going directly to your lab at the Fredrich-Loeffler Institute?"

Looking suspiciously into Amir's eyes, Jaeger answered, "Yes, I am going to my lab; it's only an hour's drive from here."

"I wonder if you might allow my chauffeur to drive you there."

Standing up straighter, Brandt got out, "I'd prefer to drive myself, and besides, I need my car to drive home after work," Jaeger answered.

"Oh," said Amir, "then may I follow you to the Institute, so that I may visit?"

After letting out a long sigh, Jaeger consented reluctantly, "Okay. Why not drive me to my car in the lot over there," he pointed behind where Amir was standing. "Then you can follow."

Jaeger's credentials got them through the Research Center's security gate. The driver delivered Amir to the front door. He carried only a locked, light black nylon briefcase.

After entering the front door, Jaeger requested a visitor's pass for Amir from Sylvia, the Institute's receptionist, and public relations director. Brandt didn't notice that Amir had signed the visitor log with the name "Maged El-Khoury." Sylvia observed the new guest with great interest.

CHAPTER 36

After another restless night's sleep, Max made his way back to Rosh's office. Ahuvi greeted him and said with a wry smile, pointing her finger at him. "The boss said you've been a bad boy."

In a classic demonstration of threatened authority, Rosh made him wait twenty-five minutes outside the office before Ahuvi said he could go in. When Max entered, Rosh just stared at him, expecting an apology.

Max spoke first. "I have canceled the next thirty days in my surgical practice. What is it exactly that you need me to do?"

Rosh stared at him. He was incredulous that Max dared to walk out and the next day walk right back into the office as if nothing had happened. He wanted to tear Max's head off, but he knew he couldn't if he tried. Rosh tried to contain his anger, but his contracted eyebrows expressed it. Standing, pointing at Max, he said, "Okay, we'll play it your way. I am going to forget your walking out on me yesterday, as it seems you have. Your display of disrespect for me and this office I will set aside. But don't you ever treat me that way again." This was the loudest Max had ever heard Rosh speak. Max just stood there, quiet, and relaxed. He knew he had to let Rosh vent before he would get to the point.

After sighing, Rosh launched into it: "Now. As I was trying to explain to you yesterday, we have uncovered an international money laundering operation that is ferrying millions of euros to a single bank in Switzerland. According to our analysts this is a new terrorist game, and our lawyer friend in Washington, D.C., confirmed our concerns. In the past, the banks that finance terrorist activities have acted independently with much smaller amounts of money than we see here. Multiple banks around Europe transferring large funds into one account at a bank can only mean one thing: someone is building a war chest."

"Why this particular bank?" Max asked.

"We don't know, but this institution was a secret Nazi repository before and during World War II. After the war, they paid fines, and their leadership got replaced, but the depositors were never identified. And now, over seventy-five years later, this. We've figured out the flow of the money coming in. But we haven't identified who's organized this conspiracy and where they are planning on spending the money."

"How much money are we talking about?"

"That's the alarming part," said Rosh. "To fund your standard suicide bombings, usually we'd expect an account like this to hold between five and fifteen thousand euros--—you know, just for the martyrs and their families. But in this account, we're talking about tens of millions. That kind of cash poses a threat on a much greater scale."

The challenge was obvious. The solution was not. "What do you want me to do? Steal the money and kill the bad guys hoarding it?" Max asked.

Rosh didn't appear to detect his sarcasm. "That would be a good start. But I think you will need help. What do you propose?"

Max thought about it. What a mess. He resented being thrust back into the thick of things, but he had to admit that the old feeling of adrenaline pumping through his arteries made him feel alive. "Most of my assignments have been solo," he pondered aloud. "This is different. I'd have to put a team together."

"Tell me what you need," said Rosh.

"I suspect we'll need six to eight people with a mix of skills. I need *carte blanche* on building a team, with your final approval. As far as strategy and tactics, that's my call," said Max.

"You will need my approval for major expenses and the PM's for assassinations." Rosh stood up and took an armful of file folders out of a cabinet behind his desk. He let them fall with a thud on his desk. "Here," Rosh said, "are all the analysts' reports. Get yourself up to speed."

For once, Max did as he was told. It took several hours to rifle through the hundreds of pages in an adjoining room as Rosh made phone calls. Finally, when Max was about to leave the office, Rosh spoke: "There is something else to discuss. Your girlfriend."

Max felt a shiver up his spine and the hair on the back of his neck prickling—the same shiver he felt whenever he was dealing with something out of his control. Defensively, "What about Lilah?"

"It is time for you to know that Lilah and I, or more precisely, Lilah and several agents from HQ, have been working together since yesterday. She is an individual with skills that we didn't appreciate fully when she was a Mossad analyst during her years in medical school. I don't need to tell you she is smart, strong, and athletic. However, her martial arts skills were a surprise to her trainer."

Max thought back to his conversation with Aunt Gila. This was the second time in forty-eight hours that Lilah's secrets were being revealed to him. *I haven't been the only one hiding things,* Max thought. "What are you saying?" Max demanded. "What do you mean, her trainer?"

"Lilah asked to have some self-defense training. If she continues to live with you, she wants to be able to protect herself."

Stepping closer to Rosh, almost in his face, Max hissed, "You have no say in whether she continues to live with me. She doesn't need your involvement in her life. I am confident she doesn't want this—and, I don't like your intrusion into our personal lives!"

Rosh gave a harsh laugh. "I didn't invite her, Max. Lilah called me."

Max was incredulous. "I don't believe that. She is a pacifist! Lilah would never want to shoot a gun."

Rosh gave a smirk that made Max's blood boil. "Come with me, Max," he said smugly, gesturing to the door. "I have something to show you."

They left Rosh's office and took the elevator several stories down to the subterranean level of Mossad Headquarters, a place Max remembered well. The elevator opened to a room with three doors. Two doors on the right had Hebrew letters *aleph* and *bet*, the first two letters of the Hebrew alphabet. The single door on the left bore a sign: "Shooting Range."

Max was very familiar with this door, but this time his heart was racing as he descended the set of steps. Rosh and Max continued to an observation window that overlooked the agents firing their weapons. At the end of the line of four shooters, each of whom wore noise-canceling protective earmuffs, stood a tall woman. She held the new Israeli-made nine-millimeter Masada polymer-framed striker-fired pistol like an experienced professional, with two hands firing at a target thirty yards away. The human-shaped paper target had multiple bullet holes in its chest. Lilah appeared confident and relaxed. Max grimaced as he watched her smooth, effortless movements. Shivers cascaded down the nape of his neck. He couldn't stand still, moving his weight from foot to foot, mesmerized by the sight of Lilah shooting with such authority.

Gaining his composure and looking at Rosh, he said simply, "Looks like her training has gone well."

Rosh's smirk broke into a big smile as he said, "Max, her instructors told me she's a natural. Her proficiency is remarkable after just a short time of training."

"Rosh," Max protested, keeping his voice calm, "I would never want Lilah to be in the field."

"I said nothing about her being an active agent, but it's safer that she maximizes her potential. Her training was a precaution."

Max felt the anger rising in his chest once again. "You shouldn't have gone behind my back about this," he said through clenched teeth. "This was not a good idea."

At that moment, Max's phone buzzed. He looked at the screen and saw it was Shalom. Turning away from Rosh, Max said, "Funny you should call now. I was about to call you."

"Why," Shalom said with a calming voice, "did Rosh tell you about Lilah already?"

"So, you are in on this, too? Fuck you, Shalom!"

Max was about to end the call when Shalom yelled loud enough for Rosh to hear, "Just shut the fuck up and listen." Then, again, in his calm voice, "I called you about something else."

"What is it?" Max asked.

"Since you left here, there has been continued surveillance at your condo by at least three men around the clock. They look like friends of your two previous visitors. I thought you should know in case you plan on returning here," Shalom concluded. "The rest is between you and Rosh… and Lilah." Max hung up the call.

"That sounded like Shalom. How is he?" asked Rosh.

Max was having more and more difficulty trying to keep a poker face, "Since you spoke to him recently, you tell me," said Max.

Rosh, who seemed hardly able to contain his glee about Lilah, ignored Max's statement and clapped him on the shoulder. "Listen," he said, "what's done is done. I'm going back to my office. Why don't you wait here to speak to Lilah when she finishes?"

Max kept staring at his lover as she requested a new target and continued to shoot accurately with her pistol. So many thoughts raced through his head that he felt dumbfounded. Once finished, she removed the headgear. As she made her way up the stairs to the exit, she looked up and glimpsed Max. She smiled inside, glad that now he knew what she was up to.

When Lilah exited, Max embraced her with a warm hug and kiss. "You're an excellent shot," said Max. She kept the nine-millimeter Masada in her right hand and the empty clips in the left as she attempted to recip-rocate Max's hug. As they stood apart, Max just stared into her eyes. The tightened face and narrowed brow couldn't hide his feelings.

"Don't look at me that way. I know exactly what I am doing—or should I say, what I needed to do."

Max, not softening his face one bit, asked, "And what is that?"

"After listening to you on the plane flight and then thinking about our life together, I knew you could never leave the Mossad. I refuse to be a victim and a burden. So, the choice was obvious to me and logical. I called Rosh and was very pleased he took me seriously. Once I began my training, I knew I had made the right choice."

As they walked to the elevator, Lilah dropped off the gun and clips in the repository, and Max followed her. Looking up into his eyes, she said with a smirk, "I doubt I will need it tonight!" Then touched his shoulder. "I am glad you watched."

Max was intensely quiet. He didn't know what to think or say. Putting his arm around her felt right. She had revealed another part of herself, one that perhaps he hadn't let himself see over the years of their relationship. "Let's take a walk and get some falafel?" he said at last. "I've missed the local flavors."

A driver met them outside HQ and drove them south, leaving them off at Dizengoff Square, in the heart of Tel Aviv.

Holding her hand, as they often did in Boston, Max turned to Lilah, "I'm not sure why, but I am feeling frightened by what I saw. Why did you want to do this? Do you really want to be a part of this world? It's not pretty."

"Didn't you think I looked attractive on the firing line?" Lilah said with a teasing smile. "I know the three agents practicing near me had diffi-culty focusing on their targets!"

"Hilarious!" He let go of her hand and gave her a stern look. "I'm serious. I know I had my secrets from you—but that doesn't mean it was right for you to do all this without telling me."

Lilah nodded. "Listen, I am going to stay in your life *and* be able to fend for myself. Your permission wasn't necessary. My presence should be a source of strength, not a liability. You shouldn't have to protect me at the risk of your own life. I did this so that you would know, if needed, I can fight. Also, I wanted to know I could handle a gun. That's all I wanted."

"I understand," Max said with a sigh, "but I won't let it come to that. When things quiet down, we'll return to our lives in Boston. That can't happen soon enough for me."

"Who were the two guys you killed in our building?" asked Lilah suddenly.

"They were Wahhabi terrorists, probably trained in Gaza, and sent to live in the US. We think they were part of a larger Boston terrorist cell. We don't know how they learned about me, but it must be related to my mission in Colorado. It won't be safe for you to return until I am confident that problem is resolved." Max didn't say that they were still watching his building.

"Seems unlikely you'll be able to do that from here," Lilah observed.

"We have boys on the ground looking for the rest of their group. It's unusual for terrorists to show themselves as they did. We think an order originated from a high level instructing the cell to kill me. Our team traced the two gunmen back to Gaza city but haven't established who financed them. In part, that's what Rosh was talking to me about. We are investigating a potential source funding terrorism."

Max yawned, "I'm exhausted. Let's get some dinner and stay in Natanya tonight. On the way, I need to stop back at RAMOW."

"Max, I'm going there with you. I'm sure Rosh would approve."

"I doubt it," he started, then stopped and smiled. "But if we go together, he'll just have to deal with it."

CHAPTER 37

Sylvia's face was expressionless when she clipped the guest badge marked "Maged El-Khoury" onto Amir's jacket pocket. The black plastic guest pass concealed a miniature microphone and camera that peered straight ahead from the visitor's chest through holes only a millimeter in diameter. Two years ago, Sylvia had replaced the Institute's original guest badges with special badges manufactured by Israel's RAMOW. She believed that someone in Israel was reviewing the data gathered through the badges, but so far, she had received no feedback from Israeli intelligence services.

Jaeger, oblivious to Sylvia as usual, directed Amir up one of the passenger elevators to his floor. This portion of the Institute was a contemporary building with bright lighting and steel paneling at the corners complemented by light grey colors on the walls.

After opening the entrance door, Jaeger escorted Amir inside the small front area with a secretary behind her desk. The reception area had bare, off-white-colored walls, recessed ceiling lights, and no windows. There were three numbered doors on the back wall. Staring at the computer screen, the receptionist looked up for just a moment to verify that it was Dr. Brandt, smiled at the guest, retrieved her pocketbook from a drawer below the desk, and walked out. They exchanged no greetings.

Room Two had a vacuum-sealed door with a small 'BSL4' sign. Brandt explained to his visitor that an air-sealed space suit with a contained air supply had to be worn to enter. This is the "hot" area where his team stores and manipulated the viruses. Brandt helped Amir put on a positive pressure outfit and then donned his own. Then they entered room Two, passing through two airlocks to reach the inner lab where they worked on the viruses. The action took place in a ten-by-ten meters square space with bleached white walls and two long laboratory benches running the length of the walls. Twelve fume cabinets cluttered the benches. Between cabinets stood incubators for growing bacteria necessary for virus production. The large freezer for storing viruses rested at the end of the room.

Brandt barely acknowledged his two technicians then introduced the visitor. "My two assistants are growing virus using the bacteriophages we produce here in the lab." His voice sounded tinny through the suit's audio system. "I know this sounds complicated," he went on, "but it's quite simple."

Amir half-listened, distracted by the two men in space suits sitting on cushioned stools. Facing their test tubes and pipettes under a hood, he watched them working. Their gloved hands passed through glass window portholes into the fume cabinets. Each poured something from one glass vial into another in silence.

Jaeger approached the freezer at the back of the room that contained the original 1918 H1N1 influenza virus, all the various iterations of it that Jaeger had created, and some additional contagious viruses for future use. Dr. Brandt explained that he could prevent the degradation of these viruses by storing them below -70 degrees Celsius. In this special freezer. He showed Amir a few culture plates, full of bacteria, which were used to perform the CRISPR process in the viruses. Brandt wanted Amir to appreciate his brilliant scientific mind.

For each new modification of the virus, Jaeger explained, he grew a fresh stock of influenza. It was an intensive process that required both labor and time. Amir found his attention wandering, but the tiny recording device on his visitor badge picked up every word.

"CRISPR is an acronym for Clustered Regularly Interspaced Short Palindromic Repeats. I recognized years ago in my genetics work that there were genetic sequences in bacteria that were palindromic—the same backward and forwards. I learned how bacteria fought off viruses. Simply, I use the CRISPR units to manipulate the bacteria to modify the virus."

Amir nodded, trying to stay attentive.

Brandt continued, "Human DNA is a double helix, two connected sides of a twisted chain."

The introductory science lecture continued as Amir fought his fatigue. He was confident his sister knew all this stuff. Jaeger droned on about "bacteria-created RNA guided enzymes that split the DNA of the virus," but Amir couldn't take it anymore, his eyes closing. He stood up abruptly and stretched.

Jaeger noticing that his 'student' was no longer listening, interrupted himself. "Maybe the details of the science are too much for you."

Amir noted that there were ten other similar fume cabinets not being used. The lab was more extensive than it had appeared from its entrance. "There is not much more to see here at present," Jaeger said, "but as you can see, we have space for more technicians."

It was a relief for the claustrophobic Amir to hear the heavy door vacuum-seal itself shut behind him. When Brandt gave the signal, Amir removed his bubble-like head covering and took a deep breath. Then he watched as Jaeger unlocked the door labeled Room Three.

"Room Three is for my mechanical engineering," Jaeger said simply. This space, much bigger than room two, was where we built the viral guns. There were no technicians at work here. Brandt explained that the two employees spent alternate days on virus production and viral gun fabrication. With pride, Jaeger said, "I taught the technicians everything they do in the lab." Room Three was quiet. Two long benches in this room had electronic equipment: two computers with large screens, one of which displayed a three-dimensional design. Oscilloscopes, wire-cutting pliers, metal tubing of various sizes, and electrical tools unfamiliar to Amir filled the space. Although technical equipment completely covered the benches, the place looked immaculate and orderly.

Amir walked over to the screen with the design and asked, "What is this?"

Brandt responded with pride in his voice, "That's my newest design: a gun that shoots viruses. This CAD-CAM computer makes these productions possible. I upgraded the original multiple times as I learned more about electronics. That design is for an enormous gun."

The tour impressed Amir with what Brandt had accomplished in this small facility. *All this with only two technicians assisting him! With a bigger team*, Amir thought, *he could produce a ton more.*

Jaeger then led Amir into his office, marked "Room One." "You are the first outsider to visit my laboratory," Jaeger said gravely.

Amir kept his composure, even as the possibilities of all this technology ran through his mind. "It's an honor, Doctor Brandt," he said.

As Amir stared at the sophisticated electronics in Room One, the tiny camera in his badge was capturing images for transmission. Overhead, Israeli satellite picked up the signals and transmitted them to a basement in Tel Aviv, 4,000 kilometers away. But no one was monitoring the recordings as they accumulated on a drive.

Jaeger was so delighted by Amir's enthusiasm that he even forgot, for a few minutes, that he was talking to an Arab. He explained how these powerful computers made it possible to parse out the genetic codes of individuals. The two Mac Pro computers connect to the Institute's mainframe to maintain the extensive database. He explained he encrypted everything with the latest software technology. He then told Amir that he had received the genetic data from hospital morgues in many of the world's major cities.

"When I was trying to cure cancer, eight or ten years ago, other clinicians were eager to assist me by providing me with human tissue to identify DNA from diverse populations. Of course," he said with a wry smile, "they thought I needed the tissue to cure cancer. I kept diligent records of each sample: the person's demographics, race, religion, family name, and family history. And then, this software sequenced the genome of each person." His smile turned into a grin. "Other people's tragedies have been invaluable to my work."

Jaeger recounted how, some years earlier, he had accessed the international database of a start-up firm, WorldDNA. Because the new company had thought they were helping a greater cause, they had shared their data of millions of people's DNA with matching personal profiles and demographics.

"How many people?" Amir asked, finding this both thrilling and hard to believe.

"I have the tissue and genetic profile of at least 25,000 different Jews and other ethnic minorities, and many thousands of Germans and Europeans...and Japanese, Chinese, and Africans." Jaeger's broad smile of satisfaction covered his face. "It's taken many years, but it's all here." He pointed proudly to his computers.

In what he hoped was a diplomatic voice, Amir said, "Well, Dr. Brandt, you are the professor, so it is best if I leave the science to you. I'll take care of everything else." He smiled to offset any potential insult to Brandt. "So," he asked, changing the topic, "what can I do to help with the next clinical trial?"

"You get right to the point," Jaeger said with a wry smile. "Well, come over here, and I'll show you." He led to the back of Room One, where instruments and tools crowded the work surface of the benches. In the center of the room, a large, round, granite-topped table contained multiple small, metallic gadgets in the shape of twisted ice cream cones. A fine metallic mesh covered the opening of each cone.

"Those little devices," he pointed to the twisted, cone-shaped gadgets, "are small viral guns. These are the exact size I used in Atlanta and St. Thomas. I placed each one inside a motion-sensitive air freshener distributed throughout in the lobby of the buildings."

His eyebrows raised, and forehead furrowed, "A motion-sensitive air freshener?" Despite his fluent English, Amir had never heard of such a thing.

"There is one over there," said Jaeger, pointing to a round, brown, plastic object the size of a grapefruit that sat on the bench. "When a person walks by, their body movement activates the emission mechanism inside, which makes the machine spray a floral fragrance. It is the same passive infrared technology used in motion-sensitive alarm systems."

"Of course," Jaeger went on, "if we planned to release the virus in an enormous space like a theatre, we would need a larger gun, capable of shooting out more virus more quickly.

"Do you need to use a virus gun each time you want to spread it?" Amir asked.

Jaeger had to admit to himself that it was a good question. This man wasn't stupid. "Viral infections spread from host to host—through people breathing, coughing, and sneezing on each other," he answered. "It gets even better. If I infect someone with a specific gene marker, they become the vector and spread the infection by breathing on others with the same genetics. Parents could spread the virus to their children. Members of a particular ethnic group, with shared DNA…"

As Brandt got carried away, Amir cut him off. "That's great! Where should we do our next clinical trials?"

Jaeger bristled to hear Amir say "our." This was his life's work, and he wasn't sure he wanted to go into business with an Arab, of all people. "We got carried away last night," Brandt started—but then realized that he had already shared too much with Amir to turn back now. "Has the Group sanctioned what you are proposing?" Jaeger asked, looking straight into Amir's intense black eyes.

"Not exactly," responded Amir. "But I am prepared to fund all of your work and support you. We have the same goals as the Group. We don't need their approval for what we do on our own, and I don't want to wait for their timetable. After all, they asked us to collaborate."

Once again, Jaeger noticed the "us" in his response. He felt torn. To go outside the auspices of the Group might be to abandon a long-term opportunity. But this Arab could help him initially with the Jewish problem in Europe, and maybe even in Israel. Amir's influential position in Saudi Arabia could be critical. *And anyway, he thought, our shared goal is the same.* He had already waited so long to put his plan into action. Why give up this opportunity to further his clinic trials? The Group would welcome him back for future attacks once the initial ones had proven successful. And Amir was right: The Group *had* suggested they work together.

"All right," he said. "Step over here. I'll show you how to load a viral gun."

CHAPTER 38

D r. Kneeland showed up a few minutes early for the CDC's weekly conference on new pathogens. She was grateful to Dr. Jones for encouraging her to pursue an in-depth study at the CDC of the virus that had killed four Emory undergraduates last November. The CDC's headquarters was located just a few blocks from her apartment in Atlanta. Because this was her first time presenting at the conference, she was keen to impress the faculty and Dr. Jones.

To fully evaluate the virus strain isolated from the Emory students, Dr. Kneeland had spent three months at the CDC learning about CRISPR, bioluminescence, and gene editing technologies for modifying viruses. By the time the second set of specimens had arrived from St. Thomas, she had mastered the techniques to distinguish the viruses. Today, she began her presentation with the clinical stories of two patients, one from Emory University and one whose virus sample had recently arrived from St. Thomas. There were about thirty-six people in the room—not a vast crowd, but enough to make her nervous.

"Good morning," she began, her voice quavering slightly. "Thank you for the opportunity to present our initial findings of an unrecognized viral agent that resulted in the rapid deaths of eleven otherwise healthy adults. They all died from a rapidly progressive, hemorrhagic pneumonia in between twelve and ninety-six hours; most died in the first twenty-four hours after initial symptoms."

"We examined the viruses using electron microscopy, crystallography, and the Virochip, and found they were almost identical to the influenza virus of 1918. While the Atlanta and St. Thomas's victims were not similar, there were notable similarities within each group. The group of Emory students was all African Americans and carriers of the sickle cell trait. Victims from St. Thomas were all males between the ages of fifty and sixty-five and had a history of being treated for HIV. In both environments, there were many uninfected people in proximity to the victims, yet there is no evidence that anyone else caught the infections from an infected patient."

"Now," she said, pausing for a sip of water, "if we make a leap of faith—something I was taught never to do," she smiled at Dr. Jones, "that these victims were the only ones infected at the two sites, then we have two distinct viruses, each specifically targeted for people with a certain genetic design. These unique influenza viruses behaved differently from any previously documented infection. Thank you."

The first person to stand up with a question was Dr. Arnold Bellman, a senior epidemiologist at the CDC. "Thank you, Dr. Kneeland, for that excellent presentation. You said these viruses were 'targeted' to specific populations. Do you think that these are spontaneous mutations of an influenza virus, or could this be the malicious work of a scientist?"

"I don't know," answered Dr. Kneeland carefully. "But the specificity is suspicious."

"Is it even possible to engineer a virus so specific?" asked Dr. Robert Schwartz, the Chief of Hematology at the CDC.

A heated debate and related discussion continued for five more minutes. Finally, Dr. Janice Worthy, Chairperson of the Department of Infectious Disease, and the CDC Director, stood up to quiet the animated audience, saying, "I think we should hear from Dr. David Jones, whose Department of Medicine directly treated the Emory victims."

"Thank you, Dr. Worthy," said Jones. "When I first heard of these victims, I was quick to say it was unrelated to being a sickle cell carrier." He smiled back at Kneeland. "These respiratory complications had never been reported to be associated with sickle cell trait until now. I was wrong. Although I can't explain it, these eleven people died because of their specific genetic makeup. As you know, both sickle cell trait and HIV have specific markers on their chromosomes. I know it is unheard of, but it seems these two viruses attacked victims with specific genetic identities."

Dr. Bellman, who had been waiting to jump back into the conversation, shouted, "If these attacks were deliberate, then someone murdered them!"

There was dead silence in the room, yet the anxiety was palpable. Dr. Worthy stood again, "You'll have to excuse me. Please continue the conversation without me," *thinking she had to notify the authorities.*

Dr. Worthy immediately left the conference and went to her office. Sensing Drs. Jones' and Bellman's fears, she dialed a number at the FBI that she had called only twice in her nine years on the job. "Hello," she said when someone picked up. "This is Dr. Janice Worthy, Director of the CDC. We have a serious situation here."

CHAPTER 39

The next day, Sylvia watched with curiosity as Amir accompanied four Muslim women in Western garb and headscarves into the front door of the Institute. She welcomed the unknown visitors, all of whom signed in with Egyptian last names, and followed Dr. Brandt's request to give them guest passes to his laboratory. Sylvia thought Dr. Brandt had had more visitors in the last few days than in the previous five years. And these weren't the kind of visitors she would have expected! She made a mental note to let her handler know about them in her next report.

Jaeger showed the new technicians around the lab. Shazia, the apparent leader of the four, was a beautiful woman. She was taller than the others and was the only one to whom Amir spoke directly. Amir and Shazia spoke English in front of Jaeger, if they wanted him to hear their conversation.

The two German technicians working in the lab introduced themselves to the four women with an unsmiling welcome. Then Brandt told his techs to step aside and allow these new Egyptian workers (who were Saudi researchers) to learn their way around the lab. After outfitting them with positive pressure protective suits, Brandt assigned them to various tasks. He pointed out the ventilation hoods where they would transfer the viruses. Multiple, thirty-centimeter glass pipettes stood on the counters adjacent to the hoods. Wide racks of test tubes containing various colored liquids sat next to the pipettes on the counter. An incubator with a glass door housed the fertile eggs for chicken embryos needed to propagate the viruses.

After Dr. Brandt explained his lab procedures, Shazia switched to Arabic and relayed every detail of the tasks to her all-female team. Jaeger admitted, at first grudgingly and then with increasing respect that these women were remarkably sophisticated laboratory technicians. *It's almost as if they already knew what to do*, he thought.

Dr. Brandt approached the two male technicians who he had employed for the past year. He asked them to help the new assistants learn his methods. The two young men felt displaced. They agreed to do the best they could, but they weren't happy about it.

Brandt wished he had a much larger laboratory so that he could expand the production. If things went well the first week, he would meet with Amir and discuss how to make his Saudi patron's promises a reality. He also recognized, as he watched, that his two technicians couldn't keep up with the women. Brandt wouldn't miss them.

Amir didn't wait around while Jaeger found work for the new lab team. Waving goodbye to Shazia, the team leader, he left Jaeger's laboratory at the Institute and returned on his jet to Riyadh. He had work to do.

CHAPTER 40

Just before Max and Lilah arrived at RAMOW, Max's cell phone vibrated. The screen showed it was his hospital's Chair of Pathology, Dr. Anthony Dibona.

"Hi, Tony, wait a minute." They got out of the car at RAMOW, and Max said, "I can speak now, what's up?"

"Max, I just heard last night from the CDC," Tony said, his voice breathless. "This is incredible! Based on the tissue samples I sent and other samples they received from the St. Thomas pathologist, the likely cause for the ARDS was not a toxic gas; it was a virus! It's crazy, but it was identical to the original influenza virus, nearly identical to the one that killed forty million people over 100 years ago! Well, not quite identical...there were some subtle differences. There was a unique RNA sequence—a few protein chains, like the ones in HIV. The CDC—."

"Holy shit, Tony," Max cut in, "do they think someone manufactured the virus?" Max had already suspected as much, but Tony didn't need to know that.

"That's what it's looking like!" Tony answered. "But that's for the authorities to decide. I'm sure the CDC has alerted the FBI and the relevant agencies in St. Thomas."

Max had an inkling of the method by which the virus had spread in the hotel; but who had exchanged those air fresheners in the lobby?

"If the St. Thomas authorities cooperate," Tony continued, "the CDC will send their team to St. Thomas to investigate. Their concern was evident during our conversation. They feared a spread of the infection and requested cremation for the body of your friend Springs, but I told them it was too late. As you know, they buried him last week."

Max realized he had lost track of things. With all the excitement surrounding the shooter as his condo, he had forgotten about David's funeral. He sighed guiltily. "Of course. Thanks, Tony, for the update. I appreciate your support."

"Max," said Tony, "there's one more thing that I learned from my friend at the CDC. The guy who called me was a resident with me years ago, and he thought I should know something else that hasn't been made public. A group of college students in Atlanta died in November from a strange influenza virus, which sounds like our case. The story never got out because the CDC feared creating a panic in the community."

"Did they all have HIV?" Max asked incredulously.

"No, that's the intriguing part," said Tony. "The victims all had sickle cell trait! And as you know, like the HIV—."

Max cut him off. "That's unbelievable! A flu virus that only selected people with sickle cell. How is that even possible?" Thoughts were racing around in Max's head.

"I don't know," Dr. Dibona answered. "The CDC was continuing to study the two viruses. They were exploring the possibility that these were deliberate modifications of the 1918 H1N1 virus."

"Wow." Max's brain was going a hundred miles a minute. "Tony, thank you for all you've done. This has become complicated. Please keep the content of our conversation private. I am sure the authorities are exploring all of this."

"I hope you're right. We're only doctors!" He chuckled. "See you soon, Max."

Max was glad Tony hadn't inquired where he was when he called. There was no reason Tony had to know that Max was actively trying to figure out who had spread the virus. Now, thanks to Tony, he knew conclusively that these viruses were weapons directed at specific people. The question was who was doing this—and how to stop them.

Max didn't hide his mobile phone conversation from Lilah. When she heard him say that "someone manufactured the virus" and mention the second location in Atlanta, her eyebrows shot up, and she gave Max a concerned look. Max saw this and put his arm around her shoulders. "Seems like David died from a deliberate attack with an engineered virus. I suspect the team will confirm this when we get inside."

They entered through the security at the door and made their way down to the main level of RAMOW. Entering the central workspace, Max introduced Lilah to Lev and Bina. Bina was the first to approach and hug Lilah, saying how much she'd looked forward to meeting Max's girlfriend. Lilah sensed more than a hint of jealousy.

Max began, "*Shalom*, Lev. What do we have so far?"

"Can we speak freely with Lilah present?" Lev asked.

"Yes. Rosh has given Lilah the okay," which Max knew was stretching the truth.

Lev said, "Well, regarding Rosh's nightmare about money being sequestered in a bank in Switzerland, he was probably correct. Working with other analysts in HQ's basement, we learned that one person managed the mysterious account in the Swiss bank: the bank's president, Domenico Bernard. We know that a lot of money in various currencies has been coming into the account. The flow of deposits far outstrips the withdrawals. It's been a challenge to figure out all the sources of the money. There have been several modest charitable donations to conservative-leaning right-wing non-profits and substantial support for research institutions and foundations. No single recipient has jumped out at us."

"What did you learn from the air freshener?" asked Max.

Lev and Bina looked up at Max as if he'd just mentioned a non sequitur. "You jumped pretty quickly from the money to the virus," said Lev.

Deciding to share his thoughts, Max said, "I think we may find them connected." Then he turned to his girlfriend and gestured to the broad shouldered bearded muscular man next to Bina, "This is Ivan, who we call MacIvan. Like the famous TV character MacGyver, he can fix or build anything. Mac, what can you teach us about the air fresheners?"

Ivan paused for a few seconds, then launched into an explanation of the gadget, a small gun that shoots viruses, he had found inside the air freshener. No liquid remained in the supply vial, but the virology laboratory at Rambam had evaluated the surface scrapings. "They identified some RNA strands of proteins and are analyzing them now," he said. "According to the people at Rambam, if this is an RNA virus, the most common type is influenza." Max had suspected as much, but he kept quiet as he had done with Tony.

"Max, you changed the subject from money to a virus," Bina blurted out. "We have two separate issues here, a viral weapon someone used to kill people and the unexplained hoarding of money in a Swiss Bank. You think these are connected?"

"I don't know," said Max, "I'm just thinking about it. I'm curious whether this money could have been used to funding research for a biological weapon—because that seems to be what this virus is."

Lilah asked, "Lev, you mentioned institutions and foundations received funds from the Swiss account. Do you have the names of those places?"

"I don't know them off-hand, but I can get them," responded Lev.

Everyone stood around in silence for a moment. Max could feel Lilah staring at him. "I might have to visit the Swiss bank," Max declared at last. He turned to Lev. "Lev, can we get all the information we need without going to Switzerland?"

"I think not," said Lev. "We got a bunch of data, but it's not conclusive. We need to see the books so we can figure out the money source in each country. Poppy and Scott, our ultimate hackers, tried unsuccessfully to get into their computers."

"In that case, I'll need a cover and a small team," said Max. Lilah's gaze made him think she didn't like this whole idea, but she said nothing.

"Why not take MacIvan and Scott?" Lev suggested. "Between the two of them, they should be able to break into any bank's IT system."

"Do either of them speak German, French, or Italian?" Max wished he had caught himself before asking.

Lev said, "In addition to Hebrew, Scott speaks only English, and MacIvan—"

"I speak a little German." Ivan cut in, "with a Russian accent."

"Max knows I speak fluent Berliner German, as well as French and Italian," answered Lilah.

Everyone quieted immediately and stared at Lilah and then at Max, waiting for him to respond. "Yes, but not for this," he said at last.

"Why not?" asked Lilah.

Max shook his head. "We can discuss this later. First, let's consider the logistics."

Breaking the ice that had formed in the conversation, Lev spoke up: "We can set up a cover for three or four of you to visit Europe as bank security specialists. You will visit a few other banks in Switzerland before going to the bank of concern. It will take two or three days. Scott and MacIvan will focus on the bank's president. I want to know whom he calls, who calls him, all his email communications, with whom he has dinner, what he eats for dinner. If he has a lover, I want to know his or her name. I want to know everything about this guy."

"Got it, boss," said Ivan.

"Scott," Lev turned to RAMOW's senior IT hacker, "come with me, and I can get you up to speed. I'll show you what we have already."

Lev continued, "Bina, work the trail of the virus. Who has the resources to do this? I wonder how many scientists in Europe have the virus to use and have the capacity to create such a gun."

"Why limit it to Europe?" asked Bina.

"I just think we should start in Europe. If the money is coming through a Swiss bank, we should begin by looking locally. See what we can find."

Max suddenly appeared in a hurry to leave, "*Shalom*, everybody," he said, waving as he gently but firmly clasped Lilah's hand and walked out of RAMOW.

Lilah pulled her hand away as soon as they got outside. "Max, what's going on?" she demanded.

"Look," he said, "you are not ready to go unauthorized into another country, even if you do speak the language."

Lilah looked indignant. "I don't understand why not!"

"It's much more complicated than just traveling to Switzerland!" Max felt himself getting angry out of fear for Lilah's safety. "Lilah, you haven't done this before," he said. "Pretending to be someone you are not, is risky. You could get arrested. For another thing, some people would sooner kill a Mossad agent than jail them." Max felt the telltale shiver race down his spine.

"You mean you don't think I can perform as an agent?" Lilah asked. Anger had crept into her tone, too. "*You're* not ready for me to help!" she said with a stern voice.

"I guess not," Max answered. "You have no field experience."

"But I could travel to Switzerland on my own as Lilah Fischer. That's legal and safe." She went on to describe an idea that popped into her head.

Max had already opened his mouth to argue, but then he thought about her proposal.

"Tell me more of what you propose," he asked.

"I could open an account at the bank, legally. I just need a reason to pick that specific bank, and I need a bundle of money to deposit. Then, once my money is in the bank, I will have a reason to visit it."

After giving Lilah's suggestion some thought, Max responded, "I like the way you think. With a little modification, it might work." He let out a breath he'd been holding in. "All right," he said. "I have a meeting with the RAMOW team tomorrow morning, and we'll discuss it." Before agreeing to anything, Max wanted to talk to Scott about hacking the Swiss bank for the information he needed.

He said to Lilah, "The team makes these decisions. Will you accept their decision without an argument?"

"Yes," Lilah said. "But," she added defiantly, "if they want me to go, don't stand in my way."

CHAPTER 41

A cool, dry evening, typical for early spring in Tel Aviv, bade goodbye to the four Israelis dressed for colder weather. Each flew to a different European city bearing a passport with an alias. Then, using other passports from the four cities, each traveled on a different airline to Zurich's Kloten Airport. On the afternoon of their arrival, a light, steady snow was falling in Zurich.

After the four got through immigration and customs, two resident Mossad agents in Zurich retrieved and brought them to a Mossad safe house in a residential part of the city. After a quick dinner of sandwiches and cold beer, they sat together to address the details of the next day's plan.

Max took Lilah aside, "You did well on the first leg of our plan. How do you feel?"

"I'm fine. Don't worry about me. I can do this," responded Lilah.

The mission's goal was to learn what the banker, Domenico Bernard, knew about the cash collecting in the account. Several resident Mossad agents in Switzerland had been watching him. They knew what time he got up in the morning, where and what he ate for breakfast, and when he arrived at work. They learned of the man's problems in his marriage.

The following morning, a Friday, the snow ended, leaving just an inch on the roads and grounds. The morning was sunny, the temperature two degrees Celsius. If this had been a vacation, Max thought wistfully, he and Lilah could have taken a romantic walk around Lake Zurich, just south of the city. He had a feeling Lilah would have enjoyed a tour of the city center, with its mix of classic old European buildings and churches and modern architecture. But all that would have to wait for another time.

Dropped off down the street, Lilah walked the two blocks to the Wulff AG Zurich Bank. The pre-war building was four stories high with a well-cared-for, sand-colored stone facade. She stepped confidently through the glass double doors, carrying a large, black leather briefcase containing 200,000 euros in 100-euro notes. In perfect German, which her émigré parents had taught her, she asked for the senior bank officer instead of attempting the deposit at a teller's window. She was directed to an office on the side of the lobby. The sign on the glass door said, "Bank Vice President."

To the overweight man in the loose-fitting dark blue suit, sitting behind the desk, Lilah said, "Good morning. I prefer to speak with the bank president when I have deposits."

"Good morning, *Fraülein*. I am Wilhelm Huber. As you can see on my office door, I am the vice president of the bank, and I am sure I can help you." As Huber spoke, he couldn't stop staring at this tall, curvy, ravishing blonde.

"*Herr* Huber, I have a large deposit to make," said Lilah. "This is the first of four separate deposits I plan to make over the next three weeks. Please, do you think your president can show me the courtesy of his attention?"

"Would you care to tell me how big your deposit is, *Fräulein*?"

Not saying a word, Lilah reached for the case and opened it on his desk.

Staring at neatly packed bundles of 100-euro bills, Wilhelm guessed there were tens of thousands of euros in her case. He cleared his throat softly and then looked up at Lilah's face again, seeming to reassess the situation. "Of course, *Fraülein*," he said. "Please follow me."

Mr. Huber accompanied Lilah to the door of the bank president. After knocking on the door and being invited in, Mr. Huber introduced Lilah to Domenico Bernard, and then closed the door as he left. Mr. Bernard stood immediately and stepped around his desk to greet the tall, gorgeous woman in front of him. He took one long look at her, with her shoulder-length blond hair, long slender legs, short, tight leather skirt, and low-cut blouse. She wore large dark glasses, covering half her face, and stylish, spiked heels. He noticed she was not wearing a wedding band.

"Welcome to our bank. How may I help you, *Fraülein*?"

"*Herr* Bernard my name is Lilah Fischer. I would like to make a substantial deposit in your bank. Can you assist me?"

"Of course," Bernard said. "How much do you want to deposit?"

In answer, Lilah lifted and opened the attaché case onto the desk facing his chair.

With Lilah following him, Domenico Bernard walked back around his desk to sit in his chair. As he looked at the euros in the briefcase, Lilah swiftly put her left hand around his shoulder—and, with her right hand, squeezed a perfume atomizer at his face. Then, she turned her face away, closing her eyes, and held her breath for a count of five seconds.

"*Fraülein*, why did you…" Bernard started, but the words caught in his throat. "Oh my, I'm going to…" He clutched his chest and slumped limply into his chair. Lilah looked around his office; she hoped the sound of his fall into the chair had not been loud enough to arouse suspicion.

She propped the collapsed man up in the chair and gently put his head against the chair's soft leather back. Then Lilah immediately placed a small thumb drive into Mr. Bernard's desktop computer. Next, she pushed a button on her cell phone.

She went outside his office and told the receptionist that Mr. Bernard had passed out. "I think he's had a heart attack!" she declared; "Don't worry, she added, "I've already called 144," the Zurich emergency number.

Within two minutes, an ambulance pulled up to the bank's glass double doors, and two uniformed EMTs jumped out with a stretcher. The receptionist directed them into Mr. Bernard's office. They barged into his office, where Lilah was waiting, and closed the door. Then Max and Ivan, in full EMT gear, lifted Bernard onto the stretcher and covered him, placing an oxygen mask on his face. The case full of euros slid easily under the stretcher into a special hidden compartment, while Ivan, in rubber gloves, left a matching but empty case behind on the floor. Max scanned the room to make sure not to miss anything.

Right! He spotted the thumb drive and remembered to grab it at the last second, just before pushing the stretcher out the door. Avoiding Mr. Huber, Lilah slowly sauntered out the front door and down the street. She looked at the time on her cell phone. From the time the ambulance had arrived, the entire process had taken less than five minutes. The ambulance turned the corner, where Lilah met it, and jumped into the front seat.

With siren blaring, the ambulance raced away from the bank but not to the nearest hospital. As this was not actually a Swiss ambulance, it was not possible for the police to track it. Ivan had reconfigured Zurich's 144 access, so it no longer rang on Bina's phone at RAMOW. Fortunately, no police offered to help the racing ambulance through the traffic. Once out of the downtown area, the ambulance cut its siren and pulled into a garage in their safe house. The door closed swiftly behind them.

CHAPTER 42

Standing in their Zurich safe house, everything had gone smoothly, Lilah thought. She admired how well the RAMOW team had planned the event-—and she had to admit that she had played things remarkably calm. In the garage, only Max spoke. In Hebrew, he gave his team instructions to peel the decals off the ambulance and remove the extra layer of white enamel paint. Stripped of paint and license plates, a nondescript, dull, bluish-gray van remained.

When Huber, the bank vice president, called the nearby hospital to check on the condition of Mr. Bernard, the receptionist could not release information about a patient. It would be days before anyone learned of Mr. Bernard's whereabouts.

While Max and his crew had orchestrated their mission, the Mossad's thumb drive had spent four minutes in Domenico Bernard's desktop computer, downloading a unique program onto the bank's central mainframe computer. This provided the Israelis full access to all accounts in the Wulff AG Bank of Zurich. Back in Tel Aviv, Bina was busy tracing all the money that flowed into and out of that one account. Recently, five hundred thousand euros had been discharged to the Friedrich-Loeffler Institute in Germany.

Inside the suburban Zurich home, Ivan recorded the captive bank president's pulse and blood pressure every fifteen minutes. Mr. Bernard rested in a private, cell-like room with two guards, one inside the room and one outside.

"All of you made the second leg of the mission go better than expected. You did well," said Max.

"Come on, Max, tell Lilah she was perfect. You can say it," MacIvan teased.

Lilah smiled, pleased with her performance. She had only been working for the Mossad less than a week!

Max smiled back to Lilah, and she got the message. She was glad to know that Max was satisfied. Without wasting any time, he began, "We have to get Bernard to tell us about the special account and what he plans to do with the money. Lilah, why don't you start with the straightforward questions, as planned? If that isn't productive, we'll increase his motivation."

Ivan stepped away and went upstairs, saying, "I'm going to call Bina to help me glean what we can from Bernard's hard drive, then I'll be down."

From the moment he had inhaled Lilah's atomizer of propofol, Domenico Bernard had no memory of transport to the safe house, nor could he identify anyone—other than the tall blonde with dark glasses. Because Lilah was to be his primary handler, she kept her blond wig and dark glasses on when dealing with him. As soon as he awakened, two agents brought Bernard downstairs to a basement room and helped him to a chair, tying his hands to the armrests and his ankles to the chair legs. Lilah was waiting for him. Bright lights focused on his face. He couldn't see anything else.

"Hello, President Domenico Bernard," the blonde woman said.

Groggy, feeling his head clear, Bernard spoke, "Where am I? What day is it? You're the woman who came into my office. Why did you bring me here?"

"Herr Bernard," Lilah said in an authoritative voice. Staring straight into his face, "You are here to answer questions. If you don't feel motivated to answer the questions, we have ways to make you feel more motivated. Begin by telling me your full name and date of birth."

"Why should I answer your questions? Who are you?"

"I'll make the first part easier for you. Your name is Domenico Bernard, born February 14, 1957, in Schwyz, a small town about sixty kilometers south of Zurich. You have a wife who cheats on you; and no children."

Bernard's mind spun. How could these people know this?

Lilah continued, "You might find this hard to believe, but I am here to help you."

Domenico shook his head. "I don't believe you"

Lilah merely smiled, "Now it's your turn to tell me some information. Tell me about the secret account you manage in your bank."

"I don't know what you are talking about," Bernard attempted.

"Herr Bernard, you are not taking me seriously. Let me help you."

Lilah walked out of the room. Someone reached over Bernard from behind and pulled a black sack over his head. The same person grabbed Bernard's arm and wrapped it with a tight strap above the elbow. Below the strap, he felt a needle prick him. Immediately, he screamed and tried to fight his way out of his restraints, but within seconds, his head became dizzy, and he lost his will. Bernard fell silent, and his head dropped towards his chest. The bag on Domenico's head was replaced with a helmet covering his eyes and ears.

After another ten seconds, Domenico sat up to loud screeching noises, and then his view filled with grotesque monsters attacking him. Bernard pulled back and let out a guttural scream. He felt bites all over his body, which made him cry out even more loudly.

"The combination of the VR and the drug enhancement looks like it's working," said Max to the agent next to him, noticing a sudden urine stain on Bernard's trousers. "Okay, let's stop it."

The other agent lifted the helmet off Bernard's head and replaced it with the black sack and stepped back. The screaming had become loud sobbing.

Lilah returned to the room. The sack was lifted off the bank president's head, and Lilah spoke, "Now do you feel more like answering my questions, Herr Bernard?"

Ashamed in front of the blond-haired woman, "I am sitting in my piss," Bernard declared weakly.

"That is only the beginning of what you are going to feel unless you answer honestly," said Lilah, feeling a surge of power. "Now, let's try this again. You manage a special bank account with over 200 million euros," said Lilah. "What is it for?"

In a plaintive tone, Bernard said, "It's just a fund where some investors have deposited their next investments."

"Who are they?"

"I—don't know." Bernard had sworn never to disclose the Group members.

"Wrong answer." Lilah stepped out, and the agent behind Domenico forced the special helmet onto his head again. Immediately, Bernard's screams returned, even before the quick-acting drug was re-injected. He thrashed about in his chair, uselessly trying to fight off the demons that surrounded him and wanted to eat him.

"I can't take it anymore! Help me!" screamed Bernard.

After twelve seconds, the second virtual reality stimulation stopped. More sobbing replaced the screams. Ivan standing behind him removed the helmet and doused his face with a pail of cold water. Bernard screamed out loud, "All right! What do you want to know?"

With further prompting, Domenico acknowledged the other members of the Group but disclosed nothing about their recent activities. The agents knew of Bernard's weak heart and didn't want him to die from the stress. They stopped the interrogation and accompanied Domenico to the bathroom, where he washed up and dressed in clean clothes. Lilah's blond hair flashed before his eyes again as the men led him back to the chair.

Before Max's team had completed the interrogation in the safe house, Bina and a team at RAMOW had transferred most of the money from the mysterious account to five offshore accounts in the Bahamas. They had moved all Bernard's cash from his private funds to another location.

With Domenico sitting more comfortably in the same chair, this time without restraints other than handcuffs, Lilah began to ask him more pointed questions.

He interrupted her. "You know," said Domenico, "my wife will look for me if I don't come home from work. After she calls the bank, she'll call the police."

Ivan sitting behind the lights that were flooding Bernard's face, responded, "Funny you should suggest your wife might report you as a missing person. Your wife seems to have gone away for the weekend with an old friend. She won't be returning till Sunday night."

Shamefaced, as he knew of his wife's affair, he swallowed and demanded, "How could you know that?"

Lilah answered this one: "We know almost everything about your life. We have already transferred most of the money in that secret account and your accounts to other locations. The only way you are going to see any of your money back is to cooperate. We have some more questions about the three financiers in that account."

The team continued the questioning for several more hours. Then Ivan, Max, and Lilah flew back to Israel late Friday night. The other two local Mossad agents returned Bernard to his home very early on Saturday morning.

Domenico arrived at his home exhausted around 3:00 a.m. Saturday morning, to find an empty house. He went right to sleep in his empty bed. On Sunday, his wife returned home with a small suitcase.

Realizing she needed to explain the suitcase, Mrs. Bernard began, "I had the most delightful weekend with my friend Serina in Paris. The trees along Les Champs Elysée are budding, and the streets were full of lovers. It was so romantic. You would have loved it."

"I am sure," Domenico answered, "it would have been preferable to my weekend at home." Domenico was biting his tongue, holding a straight face as he endured his wife's lies. The greeting ended, and he went off to the library as she carried her suitcase upstairs.

Bernard showed up for work on Monday morning, a little tired but ready. As instructed, he notified the Group that they should meet to discuss the plan with Dr. Brandt in more detail.

Meanwhile, on his phone during the four-hour private jet flight home to Tel Aviv, Max updated Rosh on what the team had learned from Domenico and his hard drive. They now knew that the Group had funded the Friedrich-Loeffler Institute and was interested in a German scientist who worked there.

"We have to get inside that lab in the Institute," Rosh said immediately. "You should go there tomorrow night. I have no one else to send. And why not take Lilah with you?"

Max was quiet as he heard his boss say what he didn't want to hear. "Look, I know she did a good job in Zurich," Max admitted, "but I'd be going into Germany without a plan…just for reconnaissance."

"All the more reason to bring Lilah!" Rosh asserted. "It's safe, just a fact-finding visit—get in and get out. If it's just you and Lilah, it will be simpler."

"It's not that safe. I must break into the German Institute at night. I'd like to think about this—" Max said, as Rosh interrupted him.

"I'll make the arrangements," Rosh continued. "Come home, get some sleep, and you'll leave Saturday evening."

Max sighed and turned to Lilah. "You did too well for your own good!" he told her with a smile. "We may have another trip tomorrow night. Get some sleep now till the plane lands."

CHAPTER 43

The azure sky enveloping the chilly March morning promised a day of opportunity. After five days in which they had listened attentively to his orders and followed his precise instructions, Jaeger decided that the four Saudi women scientists had exceeded his expectations. The new lab technicians' quick mastery of Jaeger's techniques, along with their knowledge of genetics, virology, and medicine, enabled them to alter the gene sequences as Jaeger had done, only faster.

In a small cafe on the Isle of Riems, about 250 meters from the front door of the Institute, Amir waited for Jaeger at a corner table with his back to the wall. From here, he could see everyone who entered or left the entrance.

The warmth of the wood-burning fireplace welcomed Jaeger as he opened the door of the small restaurant. It was after the lunch hour, and the place had few customers. He saw Amir sitting in the far corner, on the other side of the fireplace. As Jaeger approached the table, a server came over offering a mug of coffee and a one-page menu. Jaeger placed his overcoat on the chair next to his seat. He ordered an espresso as Amir lightly shook his hand.

"How are things going in the lab, Dr. Brandt?" he asked. Shazia had been keeping Amir abreast of her team's experience. Each night, she would call Amir and share the details of their work and thoughts on the opportunities that Jaeger and his methods presented. She confided that their secret plan was progressing well.

"Your women have been surprisingly helpful," Jaeger said. "They learned quickly and continue to work at a very sophisticated level. I admit I didn't think our collaboration would work out. But with your team's help, we synthesized and grew more virus in the last five days than I had accomplished in a month! I should have enough for our next clinical trial. Naturally, to grow much more virus, I need to grow my lab." He shot Amir a wily look.

"I am glad you appreciated the support of my team. Those women are just four of the eighteen experienced technicians I can send you. Also, I found just the place for you. There would be 30,000 square feet of laboratory space at your disposal. You won't need your lab at the Institute any longer. You only need to set up the new laboratory and guide it."

Jaeger gulped down his espresso all at once. Then, with his head down, facing the empty cup, he answered quietly, "I don't know what to say. A lab three times the size of my present lab, staffed with more technicians, would make my goals achievable!" He paused, "But Amir," he said, "we have an obligation to the Group. I worry that—"

"They told us to work together," Amir reminded him in a patient but firm tone. "We are doing that. As they wanted, we are on the same team. We'll update them on our progress after the next trial. They won't need to send more money to support your lab, and we won't need to bow down to their restrictions. Just think of directing your own brand new, self-supported laboratory!"

Nervously twisting a small napkin with his hands, Jaeger was silent for a moment. "If I agree to do this, how would we proceed?" he asked, lifting his head to look at Amir.

Smiling, Amir answered, "I want you to visit the new location with me and determine what else you will need there. Once you give me a list of what's missing, I will arrange it all. Today is Friday. Will you be ready to start tomorrow morning? If so, trucks will arrive at the loading dock of the Institute tonight, and we will remove everything you need to bring with you."

"Where is the new lab?"

"It will be in Baden-Baden, about one thousand kilometers west of here. I updated a facility I already own to accommodate your needs. Our team will pack up the lab tonight, and I will fly you there first thing tomorrow to see it."

"I can't just leave the Institute overnight and work somewhere else," Jaeger exclaimed, suddenly miffed. "I live in a beautiful apartment nearby. It's not that easy to just uproot and move my life."

Amir ignored Jaeger's concerns. "It will be worth it," he said. "Let's meet at the Rostock-Laage Airport tomorrow at 8:00 a.m." He smiled. "Bring a suitcase of clothes and things you might need for the first week or two. I'll show you the facility in person. I think it is suitable for your grandest plans." Amir understood that the laboratory was Jaeger's entire life, with no family.

"You are pushing me," Jaeger said, indignant. "What's the rush? It took me years to get my laboratory to the level that it is. I don't see how you can create an equivalent overnight."

"Tomorrow, you will be pleasantly surprised. My terrific technicians worked with you all week; we have learned what you need and how we can improve your current operation. All eighteen technicians will be there Saturday morning, setting up the lab. The original four will teach your methods to the other fourteen. Some of them are also engineers who will fabricate your guns when you are ready. The freezer for storage of the viruses in your new lab is three times as large as the one you used at RML in Montana. Your new virus freezer in Baden-Baden is ten times the size of the one you stuffed everything into here at the Institute."

"Wait—but how did you know I worked in Montana?" asked Dr. Brandt, raising an eyebrow. He felt exposed.

"It's on your CV, which the Loeffler Institute published. Also, it seems to be the likely source of your viruses," Amir said, staring straight into Jaeger's eyes.

Jaeger went dead silent. He wasn't sure how to respond.

"Don't worry," said Amir pointedly, "that's our little secret. I won't tell." Amir was glad to have some leverage over Jaeger, but he didn't press his advantage further. He shifted to flattery again, knowing how well it worked on Jaeger. "Dr. Brandt, your goals are attainable because of your brilliance—and, of course, with my support. Together we will change the world."

Amir elaborated on all the arrangements he had made to assuage the scientist's anxiety. He told Brandt that more technicians were arriving today, and that support people would be on-site Friday night and Saturday to meet the trucks at both ends of the move and help build the lab in Baden-Baden.

For Amir, there was power in knowing that he would have the most significant biological weapons factory outside the United States. He had it on good authority that Iran's laboratory was decades behind what Jaeger had accomplished. Therefore, this made his Saudi network the most powerful in the Middle East. There was no limit to how much weaponized virus they could produce.

CHAPTER 44

The next morning, onboard the private jet that he borrowed from the Saudi Prince, Amir met with Jaeger at the Rostock-Laage Airport. He noticed Jaeger did not make eye contact and did not offer a handshake. Once again, seeking to manage the doctor's anxiety, Amir suggested, "We can take a quick jaunt to our new lab, and you'll be back here by noon. Spend the weekend home, and I'll fly you back to the lab on Monday morning."

Jaeger lifted his eyes to Amir's and bristled at the Saudi's intense gaze. "This is all too much, too fast. I am not agreeing to anything yet. I'll make the trip with you this morning, then we'll see," he Jaeger.

After Jaeger sat, Amir asked, "When will you be ready to perform the next clinical trial?" He already had a sense of the answer, but he wanted to assess Jaeger's commitment.

"We can do the next trial soon. I have enough virus to infect hundreds with the right genes. I just need the opportunity."

Prepared for this, Amir said, without missing a beat, "Next week, there will be an international meeting in Israel that Jews from all over the world will attend." Amir continued, "It is the ACFI conference, the Action

Committee for Israel. The meeting will be in a large auditorium, not a small space, though—does that matter?"

Jaeger's eyes lit up. "A large room with a contemporary HVAC system would be ideal," said Jaeger. "Makes our job easier. Big amphitheaters recirculate the air as they cool it. This would be a great test! I'll need more specific information on the HVAC equipment to prepare the most effective way to disperse the virus—" Jaeger paused, thinking, "—and one more thing. Large group meetings in the late winter and early spring are a common mechanism for the spread of viruses."

Jaeger's mood had changed to enthusiasm, just as Amir had hoped. He nodded. "I will get the HVAC information for you," Amir said. "Our flight should leave in a few minutes. We'll make a quick round trip to the new location this morning. You can check it out and see your new apartment. I know you'll like it."

Dumbfounded, Jaeger felt torn between excitement and lack of control. It was not like him to be impulsive. He could barely process the idea of not working at the Institute anymore. Still, he wasn't stupid. He saw with his own eyes that he now had accomplished researchers working under his direction—even if they were women with headscarves. With a new laboratory and all that help, he could achieve extraordinary results. As much as he hated to admit it, his dream now depended on Amir.

After Amir's instruction to the pilots, they raced down the runway on the way to Baden-Baden's Karlsruhe Airport. The plane angled up at forty-five degrees and shook like a rocket taking off. The trip took fifty minutes. A black SUV met them at the stairs and whisked them ten minutes away to a warehouse used by the Khans to stockpile weapons. This was one of many storage facilities Amir's network kept around Europe and the Middle East. Even the Saudi Prince didn't know of its existence.

In the last week, Amir's team had walled off the unused space, painted the inside walls white, and installed laboratory benches, overhead suction hoods, test tubes, pipettes, and thirty-six fume cabinets installed, along with one large freezer to store the viruses. As Amir had promised, this facility had everything in Jaeger's lab at the Institute and then some. There was plenty of space for the eighteen technicians to grow virus and build the new viral guns.

The vast, French-made storage freezer for the viruses stood in the center of the space. In contrast to the rectangular wall model he used in the Institute, this was a new, cylindrical model, built in the shape of a giant water heater, with six doors that spanned 360 degrees around the outside. Each door opened into a wedge-shaped space for virus storage. Labels in Arabic described the contents behind each door. The pathogens could be separated into six distinct compartments, each with its temperature control and monitoring system. Also, the German would not know what was in each section. In the facility's center, they had built the new "hot room" concentrically around the freezer. The positive-air-pressure doors exited on the room's periphery, which allowed several people to have access to the viruses from various points.

Constructing this Biosafety Level 4 facility in a warehouse in one week was an enormous and expensive accomplishment. Amir proudly escorted a very impressed Jaeger around the new lab. The smile on his face remained throughout the entire tour. When they got to one inside door at the back, Jaeger asked, "Where does that door open into?"

"Don't worry about that door," Amir assured him. "You will never need to open it. It leads to private areas in the warehouse that have nothing to do with your work." Amir decided he'd better have that door locked—on both sides.

"Well," Jaeger admitted, "you have done a fine job building my new lab. I saw the boxes of positive air pressure suits in the room outside the hot area. You didn't miss a thing. But opening here Monday morning was so quick! I'm not used to making these rash decisions…"

"Everything from the Institute is here, as I told you," Amir interjected. "When you return here on Monday, you will have eighteen assistants, several with mechanical engineering experience, to help with the gun production."

"You know I'll need to access the data on the Institute's mainframe. How are we going to do that?" asked a troubled Jaeger.

Blindsided by this one, Amir lied. "You told me about that during my first tour at the Institute," he recalled. "My programmer has uploaded the Institute's database into the cloud. You have the same access, only faster." By the look on Jaeger's face, Amir judged that what he had said must have made sense.

Anxious, Jaeger felt his heart race and his eyes unfocused as they wandered all around the laboratory. "Everything is happening so fast," he murmured. "I need to complete the viral guns for the meeting in Israel. With the help of the additional technicians, we should be okay. The place is so big…I don't know how I will keep track of where everything is."

"You'll have eighteen assistants to worry about that. The laboratory will run on automatic pilot!"

But Brandt fretted, thinking that he had lost control of his lab. "I see that everyone here is already at work," he said.

"Their passes gave them evening access to the Institute," Amir said calmly. "On Friday evening, all eighteen helped pack up and move the equipment. I purchased special containers from the French company to transfer the viruses at seventy degrees below zero. We either drove or flew every person and piece of equipment here last night. The last truck will arrive today."

Jaeger could barely wrap his head around the speed of these changes. He had to ignore the fact that Amir had moved his lab without his consent because he was better off. Numbly, he shook his head and followed Amir to the front of the building. Although jetting around had seemed cool at first, he no longer liked the feeling of being taken everywhere and longed for his car to drive himself.

"Dr. Brandt, I insist you sit with me for a toast to your new lab."

Not sure of anything and feeling overwhelmed, Jaeger agreed to join Amir for a drink, with the office door closed.

Raising a filled glass, Amir said, "To you and your new lab."

Amir gave Brandt a filled glass, and he felt obligated to reciprocate, "Thank you, Amir." After each drank a glass of champagne, Amir went to refill the glasses, but Jaeger put his hand over the glass.

"That's enough," said Jaeger. "I don't want to drink anymore. I am overwhelmed with what you have done to build this lab. It is beyond my dreams. But I need to slow down. Can't we just go home?"

Amir stared at Brandt, not sure what he was thinking. "Okay," said Amir. "I'll summon the car, and we'll get back to the plane. I just wanted you to realize how much you have accomplished and how this whole laboratory is because of you." Amir didn't want to scare Brandt away. He just had to coddle him through the transition.

It was late afternoon by the time the plane had landed back in Rostock. Jaeger drove his car home to pack up. There was nothing for him to do at the Institute, and he didn't know whether the security guard would give him a hard time. Driving his BMW felt good, like a renewal of his autonomy. He would travel the eight hours back to the new lab on Sunday. Besides, the drive gave him time to think. His entire world had just changed. The collaboration with Amir accelerated his ambition, yet it also made Jaeger feel like a ball in a pinball machine.

It comforted Jaeger to think that there were still things Amir didn't know about his plans. Amir and his people were useful for now, Jaeger thought to himself, but eventually, he would need to get rid of them. Maybe, once Amir had served his purpose, Jaeger could build another team of technicians with the help of the Group.

In the meantime, Amir reclined in the Prince's jet at Rostock Airport. It was after sunset, and he had just completed his *Ṣalāt al-maghrib* prayer ritual, praying that Allah would forgive his glass of champagne. He wished he could have Shazia there with him, but she had remained in her role as a technician and stayed in Baden-Baden with the others.

Amir was not in a rush to go anywhere. He felt relaxed for the first time in days. He was confident that Shazia and her team could manage the new laboratory and manipulate Jaeger as needed. They would have a full laboratory to fulfill their mission. There was, of course, one wrinkle to their plan: beyond the lab setting, Amir had no back-up in partnering with the crazy German scientist. The two of them had abandoned the Group. In addition, the Saudi Cabinet of Tribal Leaders knew nothing about Amir's renegade agenda. He was on his own, and any further support from the royal family would have to be negotiated carefully. Amir was about to pull off a major attack in the heart of enemy territory. Neither the King nor the Prince could be seen to have had a hand in it.

CHAPTER 45

Despite his having flown in the night from Switzerland, HQ summoned Max for a morning meeting. Mugs of hot coffee and pastries were on Rosh's desk when Max arrived. After enjoying a swig of hot black coffee, Max summarized the conversation he had had with Rosh on the plane.

"You guys got lucky yesterday in Switzerland," said Rosh. "I heard that my newest trainee performed well." He shot Max a thoroughly annoying wink.

Max just stared back at Rosh and said nothing.

"So, where are we on this?" queried Rosh.

"RAMOW has continued their evaluation of Bernard's hard drive," Max explained to Rosh. "It seems he's part of a cabal of big-money industrialists. There were at least three others involved besides Bernard: one from France, one from Germany, and maybe the third guy is the Austrian you were considering. We haven't confirmed that." Max told Rosh that this group had been funding research at the Loeffler Institute in Germany, on the Isle of Riems. Over a million euros were sent there, earmarked for the work of a Dr. Brandt.

Rosh, who had been listening quietly, Rosh interrupted: "Did you say, Brandt?"

"Yes, why?" asked Max.

"I recall a report…wait a second," Rosh pushed a button on his desktop phone, "Ahuvi," he yelled into the speaker, "get that analyst with information from Sylvia Stein in Germany to come up here ASAP." Turning to Max, he said, "I have forgotten the details of the messages, but I heard the name Brandt in one of those messages from a *sayan* in Germany."

"The analyst is here, sir," said Ahuvi, over the intercom.

Pushing a button, "Send him in," yelled Rosh to Ahuvi.

"Come in, welcome," Rosh said, brusquely motioning the young man into his office. "And your name is?"

"Cohen. My name is Eli Cohen." Rosh nodded.

Rosh smiled, then said, "That's an illustrious name in this building." Rosh's allusion to the famous Mossad spy killed in Damascus in 1965, for whom this junior analyst was named, made the young analyst stand taller.

Cohen spoke in a soft voice. "I received the contacts…"

Rosh interrupted him, saying, "Speak up. I can't hear you."

More loudly this time, he went on, "I received the communiqués from Sylvia Stein, the receptionist at the Loeffler Institute, over the last few weeks. Her report began with, 'He said hello to me.' She was referring to Dr. Jaeger Brandt. When we reached out to her a few days ago, she told us that he had never acknowledged her presence during the four years she's sat at the reception desk. A few days later, she reported that an Arab-looking gentleman visited Dr. Brandt, who spoke perfect English. According to the logbook, his name was Maged El-Khoury. The Monday after that, four Muslim women began daily trips to Dr. Brandt's laboratory. The women stayed there late each day, never leaving before Sylvia. As instructed, Sylvia handed out our special visitor passes that recorded observations and conversations by the visitors, as she had been doing for all visitors there…"

"So, what do the recordings tell us?" Rosh demanded impatiently.

"Well, sir," Cohen looked self-conscious, "we haven't looked at that data yet, since we classified her messages as of minimal interest."

"Get those recordings and analyze them *now*," said Rosh. "If you must, use the whole damn department. I want to know what they said and what they were doing there. Also, if you have photos or videos, analyze them too. Have the completed report in my hands—yesterday! This just became your highest priority." Eli Cohen raced out of the office.

Max reached for his vibrating phone. The number indicated it was Lev at the RAMOW. "What's up, Lev?"

"Max, this is unbelievable!" Lev said breathlessly. "Bernard's hard drive included his private notations about various meetings. He used software that encrypted his schedule, his meetings, and his emails. But since it was Israeli software, it didn't take us five minutes to get the code from the company's CEO to decrypt the documents and his schedule. Lucky for us, it wasn't Russian software!" Lev laughed.

Speaking softly into the mobile phone, Max said, "Lev, I'm sitting here with Rosh. Okay, if I put you on speaker?"

"Of course. He'll want to hear this." Max signaled to Rosh to listen as he leaned across Rosh's desk and pushed the speaker button.

"Anyway," Lev went on, "this group of four industrialists has been meeting for several years. Initially, they stockpiled cash laundered from their own companies. Then they began financing right-wing organizations in Europe—and to some extent, in the US. They only support extremely conservative politicians. You could describe these fringe characters as neo-Nazi types." Max saw Rosh making a gesture that said, "I told you so!"

"My assessment of the Group," Lev went on, "is that they were trying to disrupt any liberal forms of democracy in Europe."

"Lev, do you have any specifics?" asked Max.

"The highlights from Bernard's notes from their meetings included identifying methods to support the most conservative national leaders. And they were not just talking about money."

"Like what?" Lev had both listeners' full attention.

"These guys discussed fomenting protests via social media and then requesting military muscle to knock out counter-protesters."

"Lev," Max responded, giving Rosh a meaningful look across the table, "these guys are dangerous. Rosh was right to be concerned." Max noticed Rosh's smug facial expression. His boss always liked recognition.

Lev continued, "They discussed methods of destabilizing the stock markets. Terrorist attacks on the oil refineries in the Middle East and then attacks on tankers that ship the crude oil. The result would be economic chaos."

Unable to hold back any longer, Rosh spoke out: "Such an economic disaster would pave the way for fascist states. And I bet you their first scapegoat would be the Jews, as usual."

"Exactly right, sir," Lev said. "In their two most recent meetings, the four men met with a German scientist who worked at the Friedrich Loeffler Institute. The scientist had asked for support to finance his research."

"What do you mean?" asked Max.

"This researcher was losing his funding through the Institute because he hasn't published recently. The Loeffler Institute kept him there primarily because he had been a pioneer in manipulating viruses to attack specific, genetically identifiable cells. He was on his way to curing cancer about five years ago, and then his research fell off the map."

"Lev," Max demanded, "do the documents say anything about what he has been doing for the past five years?"

"Not really," Lev responded.

"I think we need to learn about this guy," said Max, as his brain was going at warp speed. "Let's review his published articles and get the most recent CV."

"The CV is not enough," said Rosh. "I want you to go into this guy's lab and see for yourself what he's up to."

Max nodded, realizing with resignation that he was about to fly back to Europe. "Lev, any more info to share?"

"No, Max, that's the gist of it for now. We'll let you know if we find anything else. Rosh, sir, I'll send a complete report to you when we have finished."

Before Lev got off the phone, Max updated him with what he and Rosh had just learned from Eli Cohen. Rosh jumped in, "Lev, I'll send you copies of everything."

Lev responded, "Sir, why not just send the analyst up here with all the data, and we can analyze this mystery together?"

Rosh thought for a few seconds and said, "Good idea. He'll be there in less than an hour. Thanks, Lev. Tell the team well done," said Rosh. Max hung up and turned his attention to his boss.

"Max," Rosh went on, "the hack of the banker's computer was helpful. I'll make sure the analyst brings all their tapes and messages they received from Sylvia when they go to RAMOW."

"Yes. Sylvia proved to be a good *sayan*," Max answered. "Now, I wonder if we'll need her to get into the scientist's lab?"

"I'll ask Lev's team to work on that as well. But Max, your German is not good enough to go to Germany alone. Do you know any agents who could help?" Rosh shot him a playful, sardonic look.

"You seem to have more sway with Lilah lately than I do, but I'm meeting her for lunch. I can invite her for a romantic getaway to Germany!" Max winked. "I'll ask Lev to call me when they have the info from the analysts."

CHAPTER 46

t was a cool, clear Tel Aviv evening as Max and Lilah boarded an old Learjet for the four-hour flight to Rostock-Laage Airport. The Mossad arranged the one-way flight in a friend's jet because their fully equipped Gulfstream was completing a mission in Denmark. On arrival, light rain showers and chilly spring temperatures greeted them. They picked up a red Hyundai rental car for the 116-kilometer drive to the Institute.

As Max drove, the couple went over their plan. Justifying an after-midnight visit was difficult, so they hoped to get in and get out with nobody knowing they were there. With her ability to speak German like a native, Lilah would do any necessary talking if they ran into anyone. They parked at the edge of the visitor's parking lot. The guards' views of the parking lot and the land around the Institute, already reprogrammed by Mossad technicians, displayed prerecorded scenes from before Max's and Lilah's arrival. Together, Max and Lilah walked around the back of the main building where the locked doors had no guards. Max notified HQ that they were on-site.

Earlier in the day, Sylvia had placed a particular thumb drive in her work computer's USB drive for five minutes, effectively giving the Mossad complete control of the Institute's computer systems. This critical access allowed Max and Lilah to open any door or office electronically and for the team at RAMOW to deactivate the building's alarms remotely. The Institute's database would be cleaned leaving no evidence of the access or the use of Sylvia's IDs. Rosh's office had notified Sylvia of Max's arrival and tasked her with waiting one mile from the causeway to assist the two agents with after-hours entrance into the Institute. But when Sylvia observed from her car that they had no difficulty using the ID cards to get through the gate, she breathed a sigh of relief. This meant she was free to leave and not risk her job at the Institute. Once inside, Max and Lilah were on their own.

The service elevator opened onto the fourth floor, and as Sylvia had prepared them for, they found the entrance to Brandt's lab on the right. They didn't want to turn on the lights. During the briefing at RAMOW, Max and Lilah had reviewed the images broadcast via Israeli satellite from the special badges worn by Amir and the Saudi technicians. Still, it felt eerie to be breaking into a virus research laboratory late at night.

Max picked the analog lock and opened the door to the secretary's small office. Next to the vacuum-sealed door labeled Room Two, BSL4, Max saw positive-pressure suits hanging on the wall. He put one on and heard the hum of the self-contained fan circulating clean air inside his suit. Then he pushed a button, and another air-sealed door opened, granting him entry to the "hot area" where the viruses were stored. The room contained a large, horizontal freezer with an open-top—that was empty. Max stood there for a moment, bewildered.

He left the positive pressure room, removed his suit, and met Lilah's questioning gaze.

"They vacated the place!" he said. Lilah said nothing and stared. The abandoned laboratory had an unearthly feeling. Walking through the other rooms they found an evacuated laboratory. Only a few exhaust hoods remained. There were piles of empty test tubes in racks along the back of the counters. There were no notebooks, no microscopes, and no incubators.

"Abandoned," said Lilah.

Max nodded. "We're too late. They must have moved out quickly. I can't believe Brandt did this alone. I'll grab a few images of the rooms with my phone and send them to RAMOW."

Once he'd sent the images they continued towards the back door of the Institute, where Lilah picked up a dark plastic card on the floor.

"This looks like a visitor's pass?" Lilah asked with a smirk.

"Good find," said Max, "maybe one of the temporary passes Sylvia handed out at the front door."

Max inspected the card. With a small pocketknife, he separated the front of the card from the back. In between, he found a tiny camera, a microphone, and a computer chip, all placed by RAMOW. There was no name on the card, just a number. "They must have used this card to gain entrance and then left it here. Suggests whoever used it was not coming back. He pocketed the card."

They returned to their rental car and drove away from the Institute's parking lot. The visit had taken less than thirty minutes. Once in the car, they notified HQ that they had left. Questions were racing through Max's mind.

Max said to Lilah, "They must have just emptied the lab since we know the women visited the lab Friday morning. I wonder if this move had the Institute's approval."

Lilah responded, "Hard to imagine the Institute would have been okay with it. It was a lot of equipment…and it seems like an after-hours exit. Maybe the visitors helped Brandt make this move—but why?"

"Yes," Max continued, "and where did they go?"

A few minutes later, a call came in from Lev at RAMOW.

"Max, I just looked at the images you sent. I am sure you noticed the small security cameras in the corners of three rooms in Brandt's lab. They were not there in the videos transmitted from the special visitors' badges. It took us a few minutes to scan all the images to be sure," Lev continued. "I think someone may have been watching you during your visit. We couldn't track the connection. It went out through the Institute's WIFI. Then we lost it. Someone is monitoring that place who wasn't watching it before—one more thing. The videos we got from the badges recorded no voices. There was a technical failure, and the special badges never picked up a single word. Be careful!"

"Thanks, Lev. We could have learned what they had planned if the voices had come through. Too bad. But why would Brandt have left cameras to monitor an abandoned lab? It makes no sense."

Lilah broke in on the speakerphone, "Lev, we found one visitor's pass, likely an entrance badge Sylvia had distributed. Have there been any more broadcasts from their badges since they left work on Friday afternoon? Maybe we could figure out where they're headed."

"Good thinking, Lilah," said Lev. "Those cards continue to broadcast, but there have been no broadcasts since Friday afternoon. The one you found may have been in a pocket. They could have used that card for entrance and then dropped it," responded Lev.

"Curious," said Max. "We'll stay in a hotel near the airport tonight and catch the morning commercial flight out as planned."

"Sounds good, Max," said Lev. "Get some rest."

Meanwhile, Amir tried to sleep in the prince's Gulfstream at Rostock-Laage Airport, waiting for the attendant to serve him a late dinner. He was in no rush as he planned to fly back to Riyadh in the morning. The flight attendants had to cook the frozen fish, which would take a while to thaw. He fretted about not having all the support he desired from the royal family. Amir knew that the move had gone well and that all the equipment, the techs, and the helpers were safely in place in Baden-Baden. Just as he was dozing off, a text message notified him to look at new images transmitted from the cameras placed in Brandt's lab.

Scrutinizing the images, he saw two figures. One was a woman he did not recognize. The other was a man who looked very familiar. There were no other people with them. Suddenly he jumped up, almost spilling his glass of wine. It was his brother's murderer walking through the lab in the Institute. *Him! What does he know about Brandt's lab? Why would he be looking?* Amir was racking his brain trying to put this in context.

He couldn't think with the rage he felt at recognizing his new target. The Boston doctor had just left the Institute, 116 kilometers away from Amir's plane. This was the closest airport for Dent to fly out of, and there was only one main road that he could take to the airport. Suddenly, Amir was no longer hungry. He stood up and paced around the plane. He couldn't miss this opportunity.

Should he wait at the airport for Dent to show up, he thought, or should he intercept him on the road? Amir made a phone call and learned that all the commercial flights had landed for the day. None were leaving until 8:30 the following morning. Since a Learjet left two hours ago, there were no other private jets on the tarmac. His brother's killer and the accomplice had just left the Institute and would likely take the fastest route towards Rostock and stay at one of the three hotels between the Institute and the airport. Amir could easily catch them coming south on highway 105 before they turned west onto 109 towards the airport. These roads were narrow and had hardly any traffic at this hour.

While traveling in Germany, Amir and his two guards carried concealed H&K MP5's with several extra magazines. It wasn't legal to carry, of course, but it was worth the risk. He would need them tonight. In a rush, he instructed the guards to grab the two H & K G-36 German-built submachine guns and extra ammunition hidden on the jet for emergencies requiring extra firepower. The pilots would wait on the plane. Amir got in the front passenger seat of the rented Mercedes parked nearby. The two guards got in: one drove while the other sat in the back. One hundred sixteen kilometers—less than an hour's drive—stood between Amir and his brother's assassin.

CHAPTER 47

Light rain complicated the driving on the moonless night. The dark, thickly wooded road was quiet at this late hour, with only a few trucks traveling in either direction. Amir and his men had been driving for twenty minutes when they saw, on the other side of the road, a dark-colored Volkswagen Golf traveling towards the airport with two people in the front seat.

Amir told his driver, pointing at the Volkswagen, "Turn the car around and catch up with that car!" He was surprised that the assassin was driving the speed limit. "Pull up next to them," he ordered brusquely.

The road was not lit, but he saw silhouettes of a man driving and a woman in the car's passenger seat. Amir opened his window, lifted the submachine gun, and emptied a full magazine of bullets through the windows. The Volkswagen veered off the road, across the shoulder, and into a small ravine where it flipped on its side. The front tires spun like the legs of a dying insect.

Fortunately, there were no other cars in sight. "Pull over and back up," Amir ordered his driver. Still in their seat belts, there sat a dead man and woman with blood from multiple bullet wounds running down the left side of their heads. Their gray hair was covered with blood, brain, and glass, as was the inside of their car.

Amir swore under his breath. Both victims appeared to be at least 70 years of age. They were clearly not his intended targets. "Get back in the car," he snapped at his two guards, who kept silent. They reversed direction and headed towards the Institute. Amir felt stupid for having acted so impulsively. *What are the guards thinking?* He wondered for a moment, then shook it off. He didn't know, and he didn't care.

Trying to find Dent, they sped up to thirty kilometers per hour over the speed limit, looking for a vehicle heading towards them. They continued for another fifteen kilometers on route 105 until they saw a Hyundai coming towards them. It passed by with two people in the front seat.

Once more, after the car had passed, the guard turned around to follow it, as his boss instructed. Amir wanted to be sure this time. The small car was driving at about twenty kilometers over the speed limit. In their faster Mercedes, the Saudis pulled in front, then slowed to make the car behind pass them. Amir looked across through the guard's window as the other car passed him. The woman turned, and the same face from the lab's security camera stared right at him. *This was it!*

Max passed the car that had pulled in front of him and saw a man with a dark complexion, probably Middle Eastern, looking back at Lilah. Max felt a shiver run up the back of his neck and down his spine. The car's erratic behavior and the intensity of the man's stare had him on alert.

"What's happening?" asked Lilah. "They look like trouble."

"I hear you," said Max curtly. "I am going to avoid them." Max didn't want to put Lilah at risk. Since they had planned to return to Israel on a commercial flight, he was unarmed, which he regretted.

As Max sped up, so did the suspicious car. Max knew that his rental car's engine was no match for the Mercedes behind him. He told Lilah he would pull off at the next petrol station.

Frightened, her voice rising, Lilah asked, "Max, what are we going to do?"

"Right now, I want to find somewhere public and safe." His memory of the route he had just driven a few hours earlier told him that there would be another station stop in the next few miles. By speeding, he would either get to the station first or attract the Landespolizei. If he got to the petrol station first, he would seek help.

As the car in front raced to 120 kilometers per hour, so did Amir's car. What is Dent thinking? he wondered. Just then, Amir heard a loud siren and saw in his rearview mirror the flashing red and blue lights of the Landespolizei. "Shit!" he yelled. There was no choice but to pull over and hide the guns and fast. His prey drove away.

Max watched the Landespolizei pull over only the car behind him. Relieved, he slowed to the speed limit and called HQ to tell them what had happened. "We need an immediate extraction," he said, his voice still shaky. Tel Aviv called him back in three minutes, instructing him to go to Jet Aviation for private planes at Rostock-Laage Airport, about fifty kilometers away in the same direction they were heading. Max couldn't stop thinking about the face of the man in the passenger seat. He wondered if the Group might have some intel, maybe even on Domenico's computer, about an Arab working with Dr. Brandt.

Max and Lilah continued driving in silence. They still had another forty-five kilometers to go. He didn't want to speed and have the police stop him as well. They continued for twenty minutes until headlights appeared behind them again. Thinking it was the Landespolizei, Max slowed to the speed limit. The car behind sped up to pass Max. It was the Black Mercedes.

"Get down!" Max yelled. It was too late. A hail of bullets flew into their car. Max ducked, but Lilah was a second too slow. A bullet struck her left temple, and she collapsed into the seat, the side of her face covered in blood. Shattered glass flew everywhere.

Max slammed on the brakes and let the other car pass them, just enough to give him space to make a 180-degree turn. With his foot flat on the gas pedal, he drove in the other direction. No one was behind him. He was breathing hard. As Max drove, squeezing every bit of power out of the car, he glanced over at Lilah. Blood covered her face and hands. Max had seen thousands of injured patients but seeing Lilah shot was almost unbearable. He reached over to feel her pulse. It was strong—thank goodness. She was breathing, and her heart was beating steadily. He called HQ again, "This is Max. They shot Lilah. I need a helicopter here *now*."

After an incredibly long thirty seconds, Max was told, "We diverted one of our helicopters from an island south of Malmö and will land at Barth Airport, about twenty-five kilometers in the same direction you are going." They told Max that Barth was a small private airstrip that closed at sundown. There would be no activity at this late hour, no landing lights, and no one in the tower. A voice at HQ directed Max to pull off to a side dirt road and then head north on small farm roads to hide from the shooters. Throughout, he prayed Lilah would be okay, realizing he couldn't stop and examine her until he got to the airstrip.

Lilah was unconscious. The bullet had grazed her left temple, burning a furrow through her scalp. Miraculously, it seemed to have avoided the brain and the temporal artery—otherwise, Max thought, she'd be dead. *Good. She's still breathing.* With one hand, he applied pressure to her head, which slowed the bleeding. Max's right side was now saturated with Lilah's blood.

When the helicopter landed, Max quickly carried Lilah to the helicopter's open door. It loaded and took off in less than thirty seconds, then raced to Odense, where a small airport owned by a *sayan* was refueling the Mossad jet to take them home. Fortunately, both the helicopter and the plane carried emergency medical equipment and supplies, not to mention a flight crew experienced at treating casualties from war zones.

Amir's driver, meanwhile, had tried to make the same U-turn that Max had executed, but he had slid off the road into a ditch and then had to endure Amir's screaming at him. Finally, when Amir and the guards had pushed the car back up onto the road, the full weight of Amir's exhaustion hit him. He gave up on pursuing Dent and drove back to the Rostock Airport to get out of Germany. He was sure the Landespolizei had called in their Mercedes before pulling it over and had to abandon it. Fortunately, the driver's name on the rental agreement bore no resemblance to Amir's, nor did the paperwork state their true country of origin. Still, Amir knew that, with time, the two older motorists in the ditched Volkswagen and the dead police officer in his car would be found. He had to get out of Germany while he still could.

Amir was angry with himself for how careless and ineffective this last-minute mission had been. Exhausted from the stress of the confrontations, he thought about his older brother. Asif had always done the wet work. Indeed, although he hated to admit it to himself, he had always counted on Asif to carry out this kind of attack. Asif was a better killer. *How could I have failed to kill Dent when he was so close?* He hoped his bullets had killed the woman, at least.

Now, all Amir could think about was getting out of the country alive. He arranged for the pilots to take him to an airport in eastern France, where he could easily drive across the border and make it back to the Baden-Baden laboratory. He was in no rush to return to Riyadh.

CHAPTER 48

Lilah remained unconscious throughout the helicopter and plane flights. Max worried that the concussive effect of the bullet might have been more serious. Still, he took comfort in the facts: Lilah's breathing was regular and not labored, her pulse stayed steady between 68 and 72 and her blood pressure was stable. The plane contained emergency medical supplies and equipment with which they could perform major surgery if needed. Max prayed it wouldn't come to that.

To assist the team on the plane, Max started the IV to hydrate Lilah. The attendant checked Lilah's vital signs and recorded them for Max to see. Lilah's pupils responded to light, and she reacted when Max pinched her arm, but otherwise, she remained unconscious.

There was nothing else Max could do. The brain's recovery from concussion was not predictable. They added intravenous steroids to limit cerebral swelling. Max called a neurologist at Tel Hashomer Hospital in Tel Aviv, where the Mossad got immediate private care with total secrecy. He told the half-asleep doctor to expect them in a matter of hours. Max wished he could rest, but he was too worked up to shut his eyes.

After nearly five hours of air travel, Lilah was finally resting in a hospital bed in a private wing of the Tel Aviv hospital. Max was holding her hand and staring at her. The monitors near the head of the bed recorded her heart rate, blood pressure, rate of respiration, and constant EKG tracings. For proper wound care, they had shaved the hair on either side of the bullet burn wound, that went from the front to the back of her left temple. The bullet had bounced off her skull without penetrating. Max thanked God for that. He could not forgive himself for getting Lilah into this mess. Tears kept welling up in his eyes as he thought about what he'd put her through. The thought that she would wake up and continue to suffer made him furious with himself.

Rosh and the Prime Minister sent their best wishes for Lilah's recovery. Scarcely an hour later, Max got a very different message from Rosh— and this one was quite cryptic. In his rush to take care of Lilah, Max had forgotten that agents were in Zurich dealing with Domenico. He was out of the loop. He decided, reluctantly, that he and Rosh had better speak.

On his encrypted mobile phone, Max called Rosh and heard his voice say, "Welcome back. Are you ready to talk about what happened in Germany?"

After a reflective moment, Max spoke: "You heard from the agents on the plane who debriefed me."

"Yes," Rosh answered quickly, "but I want to hear what they didn't tell me. I know you saw more than you told them. I'm sure you realize how close the two of you came to being killed."

Max cleared his throat, thinking of Lilah. Despite what Rosh had told him before the mission, Max should have known better than to bring Lilah. He hated himself for having put her in danger. "Yes," he said briefly. "Listen, I need to look at some photos you can probably get for me. The shooter in the Mercedes may have been the brother of my target in Aspen—the Saudi."

"Oh? You didn't say that to the agents."

"I didn't want to discuss Aspen with anybody else." Max knew Rosh would appreciate his discretion under stress.

"I'll get an analyst to send us photos of the Khan family. You should have them in three minutes. Call me back when you get them," Rosh said as he ended the call.

Max called back. "Rosh, that's him." His head cleared and focused; he felt the thrill of a sudden insight. "Somehow, the German and the brother of the guy I killed in Aspen were collaborating."

"Why do you jump to that conclusion?" asked Rosh.

"How else do you explain the fact that, when the German cleans out his lab secretly over the weekend, they leave cameras behind that tell the Saudi I was there? I wonder if Domenico or his computer can confirm for us if Brandt is working with Khan?"

Rosh grunted agreement. "I'll ask Lev to look into that," said Rosh. "Regarding the mission to Zurich, Domenico was returned to his home very early Saturday morning. We'll wait and see how his meeting with the other three conspirators goes. Now that we have control of the money, we neutralized the rest of them, a least for the moment." Rosh sighed heavily. "If you are right that Brandt and the Khan brother are working together, and if the Arabs ever get control of Brandt's viruses, Israel will have a new and perhaps unstoppable opponent."

"A frightening thought," Max said. "What do you think about our next steps?"

"That's what I wanted to ask you. Where do *you* want to go with this investigation?"

Max couldn't tell if this was Rosh's version of a compliment. *Or is he just trying to manipulate me into continuing his work on the case?*

"Rosh, I can't leave Lilah. She's in a hospital bed, unconscious, because of me. I need to know she is ok. Her family doesn't even know."

Max knew Rosh would understand—he wasn't insensitive—but the boss still seemed frustrated by Max's emotional response. "Don't call her family. Let's let Lilah awaken first, which her docs have assured me she will."

"Really? The neurologist told *you* that? He didn't say that to me!"

Ignoring Max's comment, Rosh said, "Look; if this were any other agent, you'd do what you could for him or her and then move on."

"She is not even an agent! She is my partner and my future wife," Max paused, feeling his eyes well up again, "that is if she'll have me after the last two weeks."

"Max, we need you," Rosh said. Max could almost picture his boss's hard stare through the phone. "I spoke to the neurologist you called. He's examined Lilah, and I told you he thinks she'll be fine. It just may take a while. You can't do any more for her than the doctors and nurses are already doing. Your job now is to find Brandt. That man is a weapon of mass destruction. He has disappeared from his home and the Institute, and we have to stop him!"

A long silence stretched between them. Rosh had no way of forcing Max to go back to work, and both men knew it. "Listen to me," Rosh said in a slightly more friendly tone. "Take a hot shower and get some sleep to refresh yourself. You haven't slept for two days."

Ignoring Rosh's concerns, Max tried to push Lilah's injury out of his mind. He told himself that this was what she would want him to do.

"Let's assume that Brandt is working in a new lab, maybe a bigger one," Max said at last. "The analysts told you Sylvia reported he didn't show up at the Institute Monday. When we visited the lab, they had cleaned it out. It didn't look like they planned to return to work there. The freezer used to store viruses was empty. Where in Germany are there laboratories sophisticated enough for Dr. Brandt to continue his work there?

"Domenico Bernard might know," said Rosh.

Max felt himself nodding. "Could you send some questions to our agents in Zurich to get answers from Domenico? I'm returning to RAMOW, and I'll ask them to look more closely at Domenico's hard drive for some answers."

"Now you're talking," said Rosh. "Let me know what you find."

CHAPTER 49

"Thank you all for making yourselves available this morning on short notice," began CIA Director Gary Cummings. "So that everyone knows everybody, to my left is Thomas J. Smith, the SAC for Washington, D. C. and for the Middle East Counterterrorism desk. Next to him is Alan Schwartz, a CIA case officer here in Langley. To my right is the Director of the FBI, David Wright."

"So," Cummings went on, "you know why we're here. Agent Manzur concluded that a foreign national in the United States illegally was killed in Aspen two weeks ago, likely by a Mossad agent living in Boston. The victim in the case was a known international terrorist, one who financed and performed numerous attacks in both the Middle East and Europe. I would like to hear from the FBI director first," he concluded.

"Thank you, Gary," Wright said. "The dilemma we face is whether to condone murder by an American citizen acting on behalf of a foreign intelligence agency on American territory, or whether we enforce the law of the land and arrest people who commit crimes on U. S. soil and prosecute them. Our Agent, Walid Manzur, identified—cleverly, I might add—the murderer. The problem was that my CIA colleagues had asked us to sweep it under the rug because the alleged murderer is an assassin from an important ally, Israel, and the victim was a known terrorist in the country illegally. I propose we bring the murderer to trial," said the FBI Director.

"Permission to speak?" requested Smitty.

"We are all here to speak freely," said CIA Director Cummings.

"Those of us who work in the counter-terrorism business recognize that the world is a better place without him perpetrating bloodshed on multiple continents. While I respect our laws, I am the one who told Agent Manzur to keep things quiet because my colleagues at the CIA thought it was best. We must be able to work together. If this despicable character died in his hometown of Riyadh or anywhere else in the world, we would be celebrating. So, with all due respect, Director Wright, I think we should just drop this."

Looking sternly at Smitty, his subordinate, Director Wright objected, "Only the President of the United States can legally order the assassination of someone on American soil." He continued, "There is a process that includes the secretaries of the DOJ and DOD, the CIA Director, who evaluate candidates proposed for execution. A recommendation then goes to the President for approval or not. The victim is not an American citizen. But we can't let an agent of a foreign power murder him! Even if they arrive illegally, everybody in the US is entitled to equal protection under the law."

Cummings rolled his eyes before he spoke, "Thank you for enlightening us," he said, trying to contain his sarcasm. "With that in mind, I think everybody here would have been satisfied if the President had ordered that kill? What if we run it backward and ask the President, and the DOJ and DOD, after the fact, if they would approve this assassination?"

"I'd have to think about that one," responded Director Wright. "Would condoning a murder after the fact make sense if the victim were an ordinary civilian, however despicable he might be? I think not."

"Director Wright, may I ask you a question?" asked CIA case officer Alan Schwartz. "If one of our own CIA officers had killed the terrorist, would you be here questioning it?"

Turning bright red at the subtle insult thrown his way, Director Wright roared back, "For any murder on U. S. soil, the FBI may be called in to solve the case. If a CIA officer killed an American citizen, especially on U. S. soil, we would prosecute the murderer for his actions."

Alan Schwartz continued, unrelenting, "In all cases where the CIA plans to terminate an enemy and identifies such a target, the agency elicits the President's support and goes through the complete process for approval of an assassination. Director Wright, I realize that it's hypothetical. Still, we all could imagine that if an agent accidentally came upon a wanted terrorist, the agent might have to kill without seeking permission. Would you have approved such an action?"

"Look, we are not talking about a hypothetical," Wright continued. "A man was killed in Colorado. We have identified the likely murderer." Wright looked around, realizing he had lost the battle. Got up to leave as he caught Cummings' eye.

"Thank you, everybody, for coming," Cummings said before turning to Wright. "David, could you wait a minute for another question?" Everyone else left, and Wright remained behind, refusing to make eye contact with Cummings.

After the door was closed and the two directors were alone, Cummings said, "David, I respect your position in this discussion, and I guess we just have to agree to disagree."

Quietly, Wright responded, "Thank you."

"But I need your help on another issue," Cummings continued, "on March 8, two Arab gunmen tried to kill the alleged assassin, Dr. Dent, and his girlfriend in their apartment in Boston. An anonymous tip informed our agency that the Arab gunmen shot the concierge. He's going to be fine, but my sources tell me that the two gunmen have disappeared. So if they were killed, we can't find the bodies. I know the local police investigated, but I guess they dropped the case, finding no suspects, no weapons, the concierge the only witness, and no bodies."

"What about Dent?" asked Wright.

"The Boston Police interviewed him at the scene, but he has since disappeared along with his girlfriend. His office told us they are both alive and well and hiding out for their safety. Do you think the FBI can look into this?" Cummings requested.

Troubled with what he had just learned, Wright was now more attentive. "I am surprised I haven't heard about this. Perhaps the Boston police saw it as a random attempted murder of the concierge. I'll contact the Boston SAC to catch up. If your anonymous resource shares any more information, please send that along."

"Thank you, David," said Cummings as they shook hands and went their separate ways.

On the way back to his office, Director Wright found Smitty, and they called Agent Manzur together.

Smitty spoke first, "Hi, Wally, is this a good time to speak privately?"

"Sure, Smitty," said Manzur as he closed his office door.

"Director Wright and I want to update you on our meeting with the CIA. Your investigative skills were very much appreciated. Because of your work, the agency is purchasing the facial recognition software you used. Thank you for that."

"You're welcome," Walid Manzur responded softly.

"At the meeting, after significant debate, there was agreement that if the President, the DOJ, and the DOD, retroactively approved the terrorist's assassination, then the guy you identified goes free and remains off-limits for the FBI to pursue. That will likely be the outcome."

Clenching his teeth, making his best effort to be a professional, Manzur responded, "Thank you for letting me know. Of course, I am not happy with the outcome…but I will follow orders. Anything else?"

"That's all," said Director Wright. "You did a good job. The decision is as hard for me as it is for you. I trust you understand."

"Thank you, sir," Manzur ended the call and hung up. He was blind-sided. After solving the murder in Aspen, he couldn't even pursue it! He paced around his office angrily. *I have to meet this guy, Max Dent, face to face*, he thought, *whatever the risks.*

CHAPTER 50

On Monday morning before dawn, Jaeger arrived at his new lab before anyone else. The weather was cold for a spring day. Minimal snow remained on the grounds of the isolated building. As he looked around the place, Jaeger was beside himself. He pridefully strutted around his new lab, thinking, *This whole lab is mine, and I got it because of my brilliance! Soon, the world will learn to respect my genius.*

For the last week, Jaeger had been expanding his agenda. He figured if he had more virus to release, why not strike with a "broader brush?" He had plenty of genetic samples—not just from Jews but from Palestinians and other Arab peoples living in and around Israel. Why not infect them as well? This was a region where it was safe to experiment. During the past week, Jaeger secretly generated more virus and added it to the "Israel mix" that Shazia's team grew. It was just a matter of synthesizing the additional strains and blending them without the technicians noticing. Jaeger assured himself that would not be an issue, as he alone prepared the final virus stock for the guns.

Around 8:00 a.m., the technicians arrived and immediately went to work. Their work ethic amazed Jaeger, as did how well Shazia had prepared them for their tasks.

For this project, Jaeger showed Shazia how to alter the flu virus to be more virulent, making people die faster. Brandt couldn't predict how long his strain of influenza would survive and continue to mutate as it spread by people coughing, sneezing, and shaking hands. Once he got the virus out into the world, human interactions would take care of the rest.

That night, two Federal Express trucks appeared outside the back entrance of the converted warehouse, part of which was now a level-four biosafety laboratory. Four boxes, each labeled as containing a commercial air conditioner, held the four cone-shaped viral guns. Coffee-cup-sized vials, which were cooled in transport containers, stored the virus. Although bulky, each box weighed only sixty pounds, meaning that it was light enough for one man to lift. One truck headed two hours east to Frankfurt's Airport, and the other truck six hours west to Charles de Gaulle Airport in Paris. The delivery men noted with surprise that the contents were relatively light for large air conditioners, but it wasn't their job to ask questions. Once Shazia had been assured that the packages would make the evening's cargo flight, she made a call to Amir.

"The packages are on their way," was the brief message Shazia left on his burner phone. When Amir received that message, using a different disposable mobile phone, he called a baggage handler living in East Jerusalem, one of many men Asif had recruited almost a year earlier.

Amir conveyed the necessary message to the man in Tel Aviv and then sat in his airplane headed to eastern France, despairing. He had a lot on his plate. The Prince had never returned his call, which made him worry that he may have lost the royal family's support. Even more worrisome were the details of the upcoming clinical trial in Israel. Shazia was the only one able to comfort him. She had assured him that her team had mastered the methodology for modifying and growing the viruses. They wouldn't need Brandt going forward. At least there was that!

With the attack in Tel Aviv set, Amir could focus on what would follow. Shazia already approved the next plan. Without involving Jaeger, the team of Saudi scientists had begun the alteration in virus production that would—Amir hoped—make his next attack surpass the worst fears of western civilization.

CHAPTER 51

Late at night two young men sat on the edge of their adjacent twin beds in their postage-stamp-sized apartment. Rayan had just ended his mobile phone call. Speaking in Arabic, Rayan told his friend Jafar, "Tomorrow morning, the packages arrive. He told me which two flights to check." There was a hint of trepidation in his voice.

"My friend, Allah has chosen us for this," Jafar answered. "I can't believe it's finally upon us!"

"Finding those packages and taking them from the unloading area won't be as easy as he outlined," Rayan said, anger masking the fear in his tone. "I doubt he ever worked unloading packages and suitcases from these gigantic planes."

"Easy, my brother," Jafar said, trying to calm him. "We will do this. Just keep the faith. We spent six months training to make jihad. And we've been living in this shitty East Jerusalem dump—so that we could work at the airport. We knew the day would come for us to serve. Our time is now."

"That's easy for you to say. You have no family," said Rayan.

"There you go again," said Jafar. "We've been together for almost a year, and you keep reminding me of that. Just because you have a wife and son doesn't mean that my commitment to Allah is any less than yours."

"No, but our sacrifices are different," Rayan answered softly. "I have already been away from my wife for too long. I'm not sure I want to do this anymore."

"We've pledged our commitment to Islam and Allah. When the other brother recruited us, we didn't know when we would be called. We finally have a mission, and there are no bombs. So, why are you questioning it now?" asked Jafar.

"I don't know. Maybe now it's all sinking in. I realize that this is it—and I don't want to die," admitted Rayan.

Jafar spoke more forcefully. "Why do you say that? The Saudi has assured us we will not be martyrs."

"Look, I want to believe that…but I just don't know." Rayan looked down as he spoke.

"Rayan, do you have any idea what it is we're doing?" Jafar asked gently.

"It scares me not to know details. Look, we got our instructions. We'll retrieve the four packages, assemble the devices, and carefully place them in an ideal location, then leave. But I don't know what these devices will do," said Rayan.

"Well, whatever it is, the Saudi is very well-respected," Jafar said. "With Allah's help, he has given us a chance to strike back at Israel. So someday, we will look back and be proud of our role in the greater purpose."

The next morning, Rayan and Jafar had been at work for an hour when they noticed the Frankfurt plane had arrived and parked in its designated spot on the tarmac. While the passengers exited the plane, the suitcases and cargo packages made their way down the conveyor belt to baggage carts towed by airport tugs. Rayan and Jafar each drove a tug, pulling trolleys heaped high with newly arrived luggage inside the baggage sorting area.

Jafar and Rayan spotted the special packages from the Frankfurt flight and slipped them under the large sorting counter. They had asked about the morning's flight from Paris and were told it had never arrived. In fact, because of engine trouble, it had never taken off.

After emptying the baggage carts, both men placed the packages back on one of the airport tugs, and together they drove it around back to the service area for motorized equipment. Tools and power equipment filled the workspace. Their supervisor stopped them as they lifted the two large packages.

Speaking in Hebrew, which both Jafar and Rayan understood, the supervisor demanded, "What are you doing with those packages?"

After signaling to Jafar, Rayan answered the supervisor: "Look at this. These are our packages. See the address over here," he pointed, directing the unwary supervisor's attention to the package and away from Jafar. As the supervisor got closer and leaned over to look down at the box, Jafar emerged from behind him with a tire iron in his hand and struck the man on the head.

The supervisor collapsed to the ground, knocked out and bleeding from a scalp wound at the back of his head. Rayan gave Jafar a look, half-critical, half-stunned. "You could have killed him with that hit," he muttered in Arabic. Then, "Let's get out of here."

The two baggage handlers left the service area with two packages and made their way out a back door with a disabled alarm. It was early morning as they exited through a gate in the perimeter fence. They had planned to use this exit as it was not accessible to the public, and there was minimal surveillance in this remote part of the airport. Their borrowed pickup truck waited for them just outside the gate.

Once they had driven away in haste, Jafar looked over at Rayan in the driver's seat and said, "I don't know what to do about the other packages. Maybe we should return later tonight if the Paris flight comes in. I am sure they'll store them with the abandoned packages."

"We can't go back," insisted Rayan. "Are you crazy? After we nearly killed the supervisor, they'll be looking for us! So, the moment we complete our mission, we're heading home to Jordan."

While driving towards Jerusalem, fifty-five kilometers away, Rayan said, "Call the Saudi and tell him only one plane arrived."

"Me?" Jafar said quizzically. "You're better at speaking to him. You call him."

"*As-salamu alaykum*," said Rayan when Amir answered the phone. "We have a problem, sir. Only one plane had arrived."

Ready to explode, Amir shouted, "What? How could that be?" Amir clenched his teeth, holding back his rage, and took a deep breath calming himself. "The two devices you have should be sufficient. Did you have any difficulty retrieving the packages?"

Rayan responded, with a delay, "Uh, no problem, sir." His mind bulged with the image of the man getting hit over the head with the tire iron and crumpling to the ground.

Amir immediately heard the tension in his voice but let it go. "Fine," said Amir. "With only two devices, you only need to find two locations for their placement. Just stick to the plan and let me know how things go."

Rayan felt a surge of relief when Amir ended the call. Thoughts were circling rapidly in his brain, but he wouldn't discuss them with Jafar just yet. The two men drove home to their East Jerusalem apartment, satisfied that they had completed the plan's first step.

Jafar opened the first package in their unfurnished room on the third story of the grim concrete apartment building. He said, "Now I see why the Saudi insisted on us having a DVD player." Rayan opened the second package, finding a similar device and two envelopes. "Here are the instructions," as he placed the disk into the DVD player.

After reviewing the DVD twice, the two men looked at each other. "This won't be difficult," said Jafar. He held up the small, cold package. He reviewed the instructions aloud. "All we have to do is open the tops and screw one vial into the bottom of each device—right?"

"Yes, but we don't connect the vials until the last minute," Rayan said didactically. "As for these envelopes, I guess we don't need to open them now."

"I want to assemble the devices and see what we have," said Jafar. Together, the two men built the virus guns. Each device they assembled appeared like a three-foot-high, twisted ice cream cone with a box at the base. The open part of the cone, nearly half a meter in diameter, faced one side and had a fine wire mesh covering. A toggle switch at the base started an internal fan.

"I guess these devices spray something into the ventilation system," Rayan continued. "We'd better get out fast after we set them up."

"Not to worry, my brother. That was part of our deal with the Saudi, and I trust him," said Jafar. "He is a man of God."

Rayan went on, only partially listening to Jafar. "I'm curious to know what's in the envelopes?"

"The instructions in the DVD say not to open them unless Plan A fails or is abandoned," said Jafar cautiously.

Both envelopes, which Rayan held up, had 'Plan B' typed on the front. From the feel of them, he could tell that each held a folded piece of paper. "We'd have to open the envelopes to see what's written there," he said.

"We're not opening them," said Jafar. "Remember, we are only to open one of them if we need to pursue Plan B.

"Aren't you curious what Plan B is?" asked Rayan.

Jafar said again, "I trust the Saudi who got us here. I am sure it is a good plan."

"What makes me concerned," said Rayan, "is that since we knocked out the supervisor in the bag room, the airport will notify the police." His mind was racing again. "We should set up the devices tonight, so then we can drive right home to Jordan afterward."

"Are you kidding?" Jafar answered. "The Saudi will kill us if his devices don't have the expected effect because we set them up too early!"

"We can still trigger the devices with the same, ten-digit number on our cell phones, from wherever we are," responded Rayan.

"But our badges won't allow us into the auditorium with the exhibitors until tomorrow," said Jafar.

Rayan shook his head. "I've got a different idea."

CHAPTER 52

After leaving Rosh's office, Max got a ride to RAMOW. Several members of the team were sitting around Lev's workspace.

"Lev," Max said, getting right down to business, "I need your help. If I were going to build a virology research laboratory capable of engineering viruses, what would I need to make it happen?" asked Max.

"I was wondering the same thing," said Lev, "so I invited an expert to meet with us. She agreed to speak to us on encrypted phones anytime we need."

"Let's call her now," said Max.

Lev dialed the number and welcomed Dr. Shima Simonson, the Chief Virologist at Rambam Medical Center, on speakerphone: "Good morning, Dr. Simonson! Thank you for taking the time to speak with us," said Lev. "As I was telling you, we're investigating the cause of some lethal viral infections. A German, Dr. Jaeger Brandt, is our primary suspect."

Max spoke next: "Hello, Dr. Simonson, I am Max Dent. Although I am a cardiac surgeon in Boston, I am here as an agent for the Mossad. Are you familiar with Dr. Jaeger Brandt?"

Her deep rich voice and thoughtful delivery expressed confidence. "Thank you for asking, and please, call me Shima. Yes, I had read an article by him some years ago. As I recall, he had been working on viral engineering, hoping to treat solid tumor cancers. He had a formidable reputation in the virology world. Still, he fell off the academic radar screen and hasn't published or made international presentations in the last five years. He may have attended the international meeting in Atlanta last fall, but he didn't speak."

"Yes, and we know he has recently left the Loeffler Institute, but we are not sure where he moved to continue his work with viruses. We're trying to find the location of his new research facility. We also wanted to ask you: if he built a whole new laboratory, what would be the requirements, in terms of equipment and technology?"

"First, I can't imagine any of the top viral research facilities stopping or putting aside their work voluntarily, let alone in such a sudden way!" Dr. Simonson exclaimed. "These researchers are too protective and too private to allow such a thing to happen. If he had unlimited resources, building a new center would be more attractive to avoid oversight."

Dr. Simonson continued, "The big-ticket items to build such a facility include high-powered computers with CAD-CAM capability, an electron microscope, incubators for the chicken eggs and their embryos—all with micro temperature controls—and, of course, a freezer to store viruses at low temperatures. But experienced laboratory technicians are hard to find. Also, you would need a spacious building to allow people to move freely and carefully in handling the viruses during production. Each technician or scientist needs his or her own space."

"How large are we talking about?" asked Lev.

"It depends on the production capacity, but an average size laboratory is 1200 to 2400 square meters; some are as large as 4500 square meters to house all the equipment. A facility like this has to be functioning with a level four biosystems safety degree of containment for severe contagions, which means an advanced HVAC system."

"Thank you, Shima," said Max. "I have just a few follow-up questions. Can you describe in more detail the incubators and the storage freezer? How big are they?"

The virologist described the equipment in extreme detail, then added, "Any facility operating at this level must have at least one vault or freezer to store the viruses. While there are three manufacturers globally, France makes the best ones, just outside of Paris."

Lev turned to Max and said over the speakerphone, "Dr. Simonson, that is critical information. First we have to identify all the laboratories in Germany where they have these items."

"I think I can help you a bit more," the doctor volunteered. "Besides the Loeffler Institute, there are only four major viral research laboratories in Germany that can do this type of sophisticated work. They are the Max Planck Institute in Berlin and three other centers in Munich, Essen, and Hamburg. Brandt was the leader at the Loeffler Institute. And I just can't imagine any of those other research centers stopping their work to make room for him. It doesn't work that way; egos are too big in that arena."

"One last question, Doctor," said Lev. "How many viral research laboratories are there in France? Or in Israel?" He shot Max a questioning look and added, "Are there any other facilities in the Middle East that have the sophistication to engineer viruses?"

"The Louis Pasteur Institute is the most famous infectious disease center in France. In the Middle East, there is one each in Lebanon, Egypt, Jordan, and the biggest one, other than in Israel, is in Saudi Arabia," said Shima.

"Shima," Max piped up again, the excitement evident on his face, "Can you please tell us more about the laboratory in Saudi Arabia?"

"I know little about it," she answered, "only that it's in Riyadh. They have produced a respectable number of publications in virology. After Israel, the Riyadh center has the most experience in the Middle East."

"Thank you again, Shima. You have been extremely helpful," said Lev. He hung up and noticed Bina and two other members of his RAMOW team had gathered around their conversation.

"Next steps?" Lev asked them.

Max spoke, "Rosh told us that we have assurance from Sylvia that Brandt's lab didn't move elsewhere in the building. During her four years at the Institute, all the laboratory moves had occurred during work hours, Monday through Friday—and we know that this happened over the weekend. We need to check out all four research centers in Germany to see if there have been any recent administrative changes in their programs. If we identify the French manufacturer of the freezers, maybe they can tell us if they sold any recently."

CHAPTER 53

After yesterday's phone call with Altman, Gustav was fired up to confront Domenico. *Too bad*, thought Gustav; he'd always liked the Swiss banker—but if Bernard had screwed up, he was a dead man.

Gustav exited his private jet after landing in Kloten, ten kilometers from downtown Zurich. A black Mercedes with two security guards met him. "Welcome to Zurich, Herr Schröder," said one of the guards in German as he opened the back door for Gustav. "I trust the flight was easy for you."

"Yes," Gustav responded curtly. "Take me first to the Wulff AG Zurich Bank."

"Yes, sir," responded the driver.

Gustav called the bank en route to speak to Domenico Bernard.

"Hello, Gustav," the familiar voice said. Bernard wasn't prepared for this. As soon as he had heard Gustav's voice, Domenico was seized with anxiety and perspired profusely, thinking, *how to postpone this confrontation?* He was too scared to do what the Israelis had demanded of him. "I heard you called earlier," Bernard said sheepishly. "I was hoping we could meet, maybe tomorrow, to discuss a few things."

Increasingly outraged, Gustav said, "I went online to find that most of our money was no longer in your bank. Where is it? Domenico, where the fuck is our money!" Gustav didn't wait for an answer. "You said you wanted a meeting. How about right now?" Gustav demanded.

"I am quite busy today, but you could stop by tonight or tomorrow—" Bernard said.

"Domenico, I'm parked out front of your fucking bank right now." Gustav ordered, "Join me for a late lunch." It was not a question.

The bank president's hands puddled with sweat, and his throat became dry. There was no way out. He hoped the Israelis were watching him and would protect him if needed, but he wasn't sure. Dazed, he told his staff that he was heading out for a meeting. They barely noticed when he left.

He walked out the bank's front door, the same door the fake EMTs had carried him through on a stretcher just four days earlier. Bernard saw the Mercedes SUV with darkened windows, and his body trembled with fear. A young, muscular man sitting in the front passenger seat stepped out and held the back door open for Domenico.

Wearing dark glasses, two men sat across the street in a late-model black Porsche Panamera. Unbeknownst to Domenico, these two Mossad agents were watching him and listening to his phone. If the Porsche had to move, a second team was nearby and would arrive as backup.

Bernard's insides lurched as Gustav's black Mercedes SUV drove away. He felt nauseous. The Panamera was facing the opposite direction, but as the SUV pulled out, the Mossad's car raced to the corner and made a quick right turn. Back in Tel Aviv, headquarters was also tracking Domenico with his phone's GPS. The Mossad agents were alerted when Gustav's SUV turned. The Panamera made two more right turns and then a left and found itself about eight car lengths behind Gustav's Mercedes.

"Domenico, what's going on?" asked Gustav in a very controlled and precise tone. "Why did you call for an urgent meeting of the Group? No— wait before you answer that question— where is our money?"

Domenico could barely breathe, but he remembered what the Israelis had instructed him to say in response to this inevitable query. "Gustav," he said, trying to sound calm, "I had to move the money around and limit access. On Friday, I learned from a friend in the State Secretariat for International Financial Matters that a special banking investigation unit just started looking at the account with our cash. They allege that money was transferred into our bank without proper accounting establishing provenance..." Domenico was rambling. He felt sure that Gustav could see the sweat breaking out on his brow.

"You know how sensitive they are to any suspicion of money laundering and potential tax evasion for citizens of other countries," he went on. "So, I moved the money into five different accounts, each in a different country: several in the Caribbean Islands, one in Israel, and one each in Amsterdam and Brussels. I had to make the cash appear to disappear, and I think I did! I can give you read-only access to the accounts." Noticing Gustav's angrily raised eyebrow, he added, "Since I had to rush to set up the accounts, I didn't have time to get each of Group's electronic signatures. I wanted to have a meeting to inform the group."

Gustav thought the story sounded too incredible, but he knew whom to call to verify what Domenico had said about the investigation. He would text his contact and get an answer by the time they finished lunch. For now, he said nothing except, "Let's eat." Gustav told his driver to take them to Rämistrasse 4. "My favorite restaurant in Zurich, Kronenhalle," he explained. "I called ahead to tell them we'd be coming."

The Mossad agents in the Porsche drove by the restaurant slowly. They figured Domenico was safe for now, but maybe if they had lunch in Kronenhalle as well, they could monitor things. Both agents were German-speaking: one was a younger man who spoke the language with a Russian accent, while the older one a Swiss-born Israeli. They had decided the older man would do all the talking. They entered and sat far from Gustav and Domenico's table but close to the restroom, just in case Gustav used the facilities.

Schröder didn't go to the restroom until he had ordered his meal. Being a proper gentleman, Gustav placed his suit jacket on a hook before entering the bathroom and closed its door. It took the agent just forty-five seconds to discover that Gustav kept his phone with him and not in his suit jacket. So, the younger agent planted the eavesdropping bug in Gustav's coat pocket—the next best thing, he figured.

Gustav deliberately didn't mention a thing about the money once he sat back down. He wanted Domenico to relax, and besides, Gustav was waiting to hear from his nephew, who worked in the State Secretariat. He could tell that Domenico was not himself. And although he had always had a fondness for the Swiss man, Gustav trusted no one. He let his napkin drop to the floor. As he bent down to retrieve it, he placed a nearly invisible tiny dark blue tracker carefully under Domenico's trouser cuff. Gustav then sat up to ponder Domenico. He didn't know that all that remained of their 250 million euros was 50,000—nor did he know that the Mossad now controlled the entire fortune in five different accounts. Domenico's story was not a total lie. The only difference between the version he'd told Gustav and the truth was that the Group had lost access to its money.

Meanwhile, Gustav's two bodyguards sat patiently and attentively in their car in front of Kronenhalle. They didn't pay any attention to the two men who had gotten out of the Panamera and entered the restaurant. Well-dressed men and Porsches were common in this part of Zurich.

When Domenico got up to go to the bathroom, Gustav looked at a new text message informing him there was no secret investigation of the Wulff Bank accounts. With that information, Gustav smiled a crafty smirk and lifted his cell phone and spoke to the two guards in his car.

Gustav greeted Domenico as he returned to the table. The two men finished their lunch in awkward silence. After the meal, Gustav accompanied Domenico back into the SUV. Before getting into his car, signaling to his companion that he had to take a call, Gustav used his phone to send a message.

Still in the restaurant, the Israeli agents heard Gustav's message faintly from the bug in his jacket pocket. While waiting for Gustav's car doors to close, the older Mossad agent made a call— and then made their move. As the two Mossad agents got in their car, the younger man drove and spoke: "We'd better follow closely; we can't lose Domenico. The backup team got my message and will follow as well."

The Mercedes driver first dropped Gustav off at his office. Domenico was still in the back seat and heard the doors lock after Gustav exited. The guard in the driver's seat sped up the car and commented that they were doing a small errand for Gustav before returning Domenico to his bank. The other guard reached into the glove compartment.

"I need to get back to my office," Domenico said, trying to keep the note of panic out of his voice.

The guards ignored him.

"If you don't stop the car, I'm going to open the door myself," he said, more loudly this time. He had forgotten that the doors were locked. When he couldn't unlock the doors, he exploded with fear and screamed, "What's going on? I insist you drop me off *now!*"

The car stopped promptly, and the guard in the front passenger seat jumped out and pushed next to Domenico into the SUV's backseat. Startled, Domenico's eyes exploded when he felt the guard jab him in the neck with a syringe. His last thought before the world went dark was that the car was speeding up.

The guard in the front seat drove the SUV down a small, residential street in a middle-class neighborhood. The homes were built along a hilly ridge that gave great views down over a valley. The street was at the base of the hill, at the level of the first-floor garage. The houses along the road had a similar design, such that owners could drive directly into their two-car, ground-floor garages.

The garage door, familiar to the driver, opened as he approached. He closed the door behind him with a button. They dragged a groggy Domenico roughly along the floor of the spacious garage to a chair. As he awoke in the darkness, they lashed his hands and legs to the chair. Domenico thought with a shudder, *Not again.*

His head was spinning. He felt pain in his neck where the needle had stuck him, and he had a throbbing headache. There was a bright light shining into his face. He could not make out the two men around him. However, he recognized the voice of one of the guards.

"Herr Bernard," the voice boomed, "The Group wants to know what you did with their money." The drug had clouded Bernard's senses, but he understood.

"What did you inject?" he asked, slurring his words.

"Look, Mr. Bernard. We are in no rush. Tell us what you did with the Group's money. We have ways to make you talk." And with that, the guard punched Domenico in the abdomen. Domenico collapsed forward and vomited the excellent lunch Gustav had bought for him. The guards turned away, disgusted. They didn't like this part of the job.

The driver said to the other guard, "Clean that up."

The other guard protested, "You punched him; you clean it up! I'm not your slave."

The two guards yelled at each other.

All Domenico could think about was the Israelis. They had promised they would protect him! But where were they now?

CHAPTER 54

The two Mossad agents in the Porsche had followed the black SUV with tinted windows for fifteen minutes, driving out of downtown Zurich and into the quiet suburbs. They turned into Kreis 10, a modest residential district, and trailed the SUV as it turned towards a garage, entered, and disappeared behind the automatic door. The Mossad agents assumed this was a private house. All they knew for sure was that they had to keep Domenico alive at all costs.

The Porsche Panamera parked twenty-five meters down the suburban street from the closed garage door. A long staircase with switchbacks connected the street level to the front door, which stood on the hill four meters above the street. The two agents raced up the stairs. Seeing no one in the windows and no lights on, the younger agent delicately unlocked the front door of the small pink house. No alarms sounded. No one else was home except a small cat, whom the older agent affectionately lifted and placed inside a bedroom, shutting the door. They made their way downstairs. Listening at the door to the garage, they could hear the guards yelling. To the right of the indoor garage entrance was the electric panel for the house. Signaling each other with their eyes and a head nod, they flipped the master switch. The house's power went out.

The two agents stood on either side of the door, the younger one with a long-bladed knife in his hand. They had figured that a blackout in the garage would lead one of Gustav's guards to step through the door to reach for the panel. As the guard inside the garage did just that, the younger Mossad agent pulled the door open forcefully, pulling the guard out and impaling the unlucky man on the long blade; a brief scream ended with immediate death. The agent exhaled sharply, thinking, *One down, one to go.*

Gustav's other guard lifted his gun and began shooting towards the scream, but it was too dark for him to see anything. The two Mossad agents kept their heads low, squatting as they stepped into the garage. Still crouching down, they separated, one trailing along each wall on either side of the door. Their night vision was returning, but so was that of the remaining guard. The guard fired his gun again towards the door, but the bullet struck a foot higher than the older agent's head. A muzzle flash was all the agents needed to see the shooter. At the exact moment, they raised their weapons and fired four bullets into the head of the second guard.

Breathing hard, the older agent returned to the panel to turn on the power. His younger partner reached Domenico in the smelly putrid air, undid his shackles, and helped him to his feet. Domenico blinked hard, disoriented, and terrified. He didn't recognize these men, but he realized that his life had been spared.

"Thank you," Domenico said to the agents. "Are you Mossad?"

The agents didn't answer. "Come with us," said the older one in perfect Swiss German. The agent pulled out his mobile phone and typed in a series of numbers, then hung up. Before leaving the garage, the two agents frisked the dead guards and confiscated their cell phones, wallets, and guns. The three walked out of the garage door that opened to the street. Domenico could barely walk, but he inhaled a deep breath of fresh air, which helped. Still, he needed both agents' support. The older agent ran down the street to retrieve the Porsche.

Within minutes, the Mossad backup team responded. They left their Audi Q7 on the street and entered the garage door. First, they threw

Gustav's two dead guards into the back of the Mercedes SUV. Then, grabbing the keys, one agent drove the Mercedes out, closed the garage door behind him, and followed the Porsche and Audi down the street.

One of the two Mossad agents in the Porsche spoke to Domenico in the back seat, "We'll drive you home. Pack one small bag. We'll wait for you. Call the bank now and tell them you have an urgent business trip out of the country. Do not notify anyone else—not even your wife."

"What will happen to the two guards in the garage?" Domenico demanded. "Gustav sent them to interrogate me and probably kill me. When he finds out…he'll send others."

The older Mossad agent said, "Just be fast when we get to your house."

The Chief of Security for Gustav's company reached Gustav in his office. Gustav's first question was, "What did the guards learn from Domenico?"

"Well, Herr Schröder, I can't reach the two guards on their cell phones. I have been following the tracker on Domenico. It is no longer in that garage; now it is in Domenico's house," said the security chief to Mr. Gustav Schröder. "I sent a second team to his home."

"Yes," said Gustav. "Do whatever you have to do to recover our 250 million euros. Find out what he did with it, and don't let him die until you find our money."

It was a thirty-minute drive from the garage in Kreis 10 to Domenico's circular driveway. When he beheld the palatial home with a large driveway and surrounding steel fence, the younger agent commented wryly, "Looks like I should have been a banker!" He accompanied Domenico inside while the older agent stayed in the car.

Five minutes later, a black BMW SUV passed in front of the long driveway. The older agent in the Porsche saw the SUV make a second pass in front of the home and park across the street. He hit a button on his cell phone and notified the agent inside as he watched two men get out of their car.

As they approached the Porsche, both men drew their guns.

"Shit," the older Mossad agent muttered to himself. He fastened his seatbelt and revved his engine. The younger agent, still inside with Domenico, directed him into a main-floor bathroom and told him to lock the door and lie down on the floor. Then the agent exited via the back door of the house and went around to the side. From there, he could stay hidden but still see what was happening out front.

The Mossad agent in the Porsche pulled out of the driveway and drove right into the men, knocking one down and causing the other to jump out of the way. The guard who had jumped away stayed focused on the Porsche. He lifted his gun to shoot the driver — and then, so fast the guard didn't have a chance to turn around, two bullets struck him in the head.

"Good shot," said his older colleague, lowering the window. "I owe you one for that."

The younger agent evaluated the guard, who lay flat on the ground halfway under the Porsche. The Porsche's driver backed up the car, revealing the crushed head of the guard he had hit.

"The younger agent nodded approvingly to his senior partner. "After we get these two bodies into the SUV, do you want to take Domenico in the Porsche?"

The older agent responded, "Okay. Drive the SUV to the long-term parking at the airport. When the second team gets there, we don't want to create a caravan of SUVs lining up with dead bodies. I'll update the other team, then pick you up at the parking lot. We'll meet at the private terminal." His partner nodded.

The four agents and Domenico met at the private air terminal, boarded a Mossad jet headed to Tel Aviv, and toasted their success as the plane took off.

The older agent addressed Domenico, "My job is to take you to Tel Aviv. The rest is above my pay grade. But first, we need to know how these men found you at your home. Did you call Gustav?"

"No!" said Domenico emphatically. "Why would I call him?" he cried. "They wanted to kill me!"

The older Mossad agent was quiet for a moment and then said, "Mr. Bernard, please take off your pants."

"Why?" Domenico was incredulous and gave him an offended look.

"I need to see your pants," the older agent said again more forcefully. Domenico reluctantly complied.

As the agent examined the bottom cuff of the trousers carefully, Domenico realized what had happened. "How did you know?" he demanded.

The agent thought how careless he had been while in the restaurant, but he said only, "I should have recognized that a man like Schröder doesn't pick up his napkin." Then he unbuckled his seatbelt, walked to the front of the plane, and spoke to the pilot. The aircraft began a gradual descent and depressurized to slow down and cruise at an altitude of 5,000 feet. With the cabin door slightly ajar, the agent ejected the transponder quickly over the Alps. A frigid wind blew hard in his face, and he shut the door firmly. Next stop: Tel Aviv.

CHAPTER 55

The agents transported an exhausted Domenico from the airplane, blindfolded, to a safe house about eight kilometers outside Tel Aviv. The house had been built in a Moshav, a small community of individually-owned modest farms and factories known for building high-tech microcomputers. In the back, behind an apple orchard, sat an oppressive-looking gray building with very high, narrow windows on each of its two floors. The doors were solid steel, although covered with a painted wood veneer. The exterior construction matched that of the other buildings in the community, except that the walls in this tiny house were bulletproof, as were the windows.

Holding his arms, the agents frog-walked Domenico into a bedroom on the first floor. The room was furnished with a plywood platform bed with a firm foam mattress. Although it looked ordinary, the mattress contained sensors that recorded respiratory and heart rates, weight, and temperature of the person it supported. Microphones and other sensors recorded the pulse, blood pressure and respirations wherever the room's inhabitant moved. A simple steel chair sat behind a table that doubled as a desk. Video cameras hid in the room corners and in the overhead fixture, as well as in the bathroom. Measuring the vital signs was the best way to know how a subject was tolerating captivity.

Max entered Domenico's cell with Zalman, the young Mossad agent who had accompanied Max and Lilah on the flight from Boston to Tel Aviv. "Good evening, Mr. Bernard," Max said, speaking in English. He continued, "Welcome to Israel. I assume your trip here was comfortable."

Barely able to keep his head up, Bernard angrily managed to spit out, "What are you going to do with me? I can't go back to Switzerland. Gustav and his henchmen tried to kill me!"

"I know. That is why we brought you here. It is safe for you here."

Emitting a low moan, the captive answered, "You expect me to live in Israel?"

"Why not? You don't have to be Jewish to live here."

"I must return to Europe. I can't stay here," Domenico demanded, his face tense with distaste.

"We are going to help you adjust to a new life, but that will take time. What's more pressing right now is the matter concerning your Group's prized scientist, Dr. Jaeger Brandt. I want to know the Group's plans for him. I want you to tell me everything you know about this man."

Domenico was quiet. *If the Jews already knew about Brandt,* he thought, *there may not be much else to use as leverage.* And anyway, he was exhausted. It felt as if he had aged ten years in one day.

"I know nothing about Brandt," he said wearily.

Max realized Domenico would not cooperate unless pressed. "Mr. Bernard, I can't believe you want to experience the virtual reality helmet again..." he said.

"Are you crazy? That was the worst torture!" screamed Domenico.

Staring directly into Domenico's eyes, Max said calmly, "Maybe you have nothing else to tell us. In that case, we should just kill you and not waste our time."

Domenico believed what Max had said. He didn't know what to do. Finally, exhausted, he asked, "What do you want to know?"

"Tell me something I don't know about Dr. Jaeger Brandt."

Domenico realized he had no reason to hold back except to keep himself alive. He didn't know that much about Brandt, but the Jews didn't know that. "Brandt had a tough childhood."

"How would you know that?" asked a surprised Zalman, who had kept so quiet that Domenico had forgotten he was there.

"The Group did meticulous research on anyone invited to meet with us."

"Go ahead, tell us about his childhood," said Max.

"The Group needed to know the politics and the person before we would invite someone into our trust. Since he's a German, we had access to all the private records of his schooling and employment experience. He was a strange young man with no friends. But was a brilliant scholar and we didn't care about his lack of a social life."

"What was the Group's interest in him?"

"What do you mean?" asked Domenico.

"Why would some businessmen be interested in the work of this German virologist?"

Trying to figure out how to answer this question without giving too much away, Bernard hesitated. "The Group had an interest in…changing the culture of Europe."

"How?" asked Max.

"Well, we supported the campaigns of like-minded politicians."

"Explain what you mean by 'like-minded,'" Max demanded.

Domenico made a non-committal sound. "Well…it's just that we'd like to see a return to more conservative values."

"For example?"

"Immigration is destroying the fabric of our society. We oppose governments that set high taxes to support the poor and provide health care, mostly to immigrants. So, we pursue solutions to these social issues." Domenico wondered whether he'd already said too much, but Max's face didn't give anything away.

"How did the Group find him?" asked Max.

"Who? Brandt?" asked Domenico.

"Don't fuck with me," said Max. He turned to Zalman suddenly and said, "Please get the black headcover and the special helmet for Mr. Bernard. Our client needs some encouragement."

The prisoner shuddered. "Okay, okay. Let me continue. We learned about Brandt from a lecture he gave at an annual forum at the Institute. He pioneered the use of engineered viruses to fight tumors," offered Domenico.

"I could have learned that from reading a medical journal," responded Max. "Tell me more."

"Brandt came to meet with us several times. He presented his research."

"I understand he asked you to support the research. Is that true?"

"Yes," Domenico responded, thinking that these guys knew more than he had realized.

"Then what?" Max pressed him.

"He showed us his results of the use of his engineered viruses. It wasn't to kill tumors." As soon as Domenico said it, he wished he hadn't.

A shiver ascended Max's vertebrae up to his neck. His stomach twisted, fearing what he was about to hear. "What did he show the Group?"

Domenico was quiet, thinking. "Dr. Brandt presented the results of two clinical trials," he said sheepishly.

Max pressed his advantage: "Say more."

Feeling Max's laser gaze, Domenico averted his eyes. Then, clearing his throat, he finally said, "Dr. Brandt showed the results of the release he had orchestrated. It didn't hurt everybody…only the targets."

"Go on, Mr. Bernard."

"His first trial was in Atlanta against some people," Domenico said softly.

Feeling agitated, Max demanded, "What were the results?"

Bernard answered, "Only four African American college students with sickle cell died from the exposure to the virus. That was his target population."

"That's disgusting," said Max. Although he suspected as much, hearing this man say it so dismissively was galling. "How did the Group react to that?" he asked.

"At a previous meeting, Dr. Brandt boasted about what he could do. The results impressed the other members and me. As Dr. Brandt requested, I wired the Institute the money he needed to continue his research. You realize this man is a scientific genius."

Max squeezed his rolled lips as his teeth clenched and his face hardened. Finally, he asked, "What did this *genius* do next?"

Domenico worried about where this line of questioning was heading. He answered, trying to sound almost casual, "There was another clinical trial we heard about in the Caribbean…"

Cutting him off, "When did you see Brandt last?"

"He made a presentation to the Group the first or second week of March, after his successful second trial. That was the last time I saw him."

"Where was the clinical trial in the Caribbean?"

"St. Thomas," Domenico responded.

Immediately, Max realized his suspicions had been correct; Brandt's "trial" had killed David Springs. He had to learn more.

"What did he do in St. Thomas?"

"It was clear from the report, which we verified, that Dr. Brandt released a virus in a hotel where male homosexuals congregated. It was amazing: he killed only the old fags who had previously contracted HIV. Good riddance!"

Max thought back to the sight of David, with blood crusted around his nose and all over his shirt. He took a step, leaned towards Domenico, and punched him in the face, knocking him out of his chair. On the floor, Bernard curled up on his side, choking. Zalman had to restrain Max from kicking Domenico. Without another word, Max left the room and went outside. He needed to take a deep breath and calm himself down.

It was not like Max to lose control. It was not productive, he knew, but David had lost his life, and now Lilah was in the hospital! Max took a deep breath and refocused. He needed to find out Brandt's plan to use the virus and hopefully prevent any more murders by this psychopathic scientist. If this guy could make a virus that kills certain gay men, undoubtedly, he could engineer viral weapons to target populations on a larger scale. Dent went back inside.

"I apologize," Max said to Domenico through clenched teeth.

Zalman helped Bernard to the chair and gave him water to drink. Coughing as he tried to catch his breath, Domenico didn't speak and could barely look at Max. He held his hand to the sore side of his face.

"I need you to tell me how Brandt could create such a virus."

Looking up at Max, Domenico responded with a hint of scorn, "I'm a banker. I don't pretend to understand the science."

"What plans does Brandt have for the next trial?"

"I don't know," he answered. "At our last meeting, the Group introduced an Arab to Brandt. The way we left it; Gustav had assigned Dr. Brandt to work with Mr. Khan in planning future attacks."

"Did you say Khan?" asked Max.

"Yeah. That was the Arab Gustav had invited. I think he was from Saudi Arabia," Domenico responded warily.

Max stood up straight at this revelation, his face intensely focused on Domenico, thinking: *The guy who shot Lilah worked with Brandt, and the Group brought them together.* "Why was Khan invited?" demanded Max.

Domenico didn't want to answer this question. "I'm not sure," he responded.

"Bullshit," said Max, hovering over Domenico menacingly.

Domenico was so tired and anxious he thought he might faint. He closed his eyes and answered. "The assignment to work with the Saudi did not make Brandt happy. I don't know what they planned to do together." Now he was truthful; he was too exhausted to lie.

Thinking that he would come back to that subject, Max changed the course of the questions. "Is Gustav the group's leader?"

"Yes."

"How many members are in the Group?"

"Four, including me."

"Tell me about the others."

Reluctantly, Domenico complied. What more did he have to lose? His partners had already tried to have him murdered. Bernard told Max about Altman Ansel from Germany, Beau Lancelot from France, and Gustav from Austria.

"How do you communicate with each other?" Max asked.

"We each have a private mobile number we use only for Group issues. That was how I reached everybody to request a meeting."

"And then Gustav tried to have you killed. I guess you two aren't friends anymore."

Domenico glared at him and said nothing.

"Tell me about the Arab," said Max.

"I told you, he's from Saudi Arabia. Originally his brother was supposed to meet with us, but the brother died recently."

Max was incredulous. "I don't know the detail," Domenico was saying. The younger Khan brother is the one who came to our meeting in Nuremberg. We were told he had a lot of experience managing terrorist activities in the Middle East. Again, Gustav knows more about this than I do. But the idea was to provide outlets for Dr. Brandt to distribute his viruses." Max was about to ask another question, but Domenico gave him a pleading look. "Listen, I'm exhausted," he said, "I am cooperating as you can see—but please let me sleep?"

Wanting to keep Domenico compliant, Max agreed. He left the building and stood outside in the dark for a moment, his thoughts racing. The Khan terrorist network was collaborating with Brandt! But what was

Amir doing in that part of Germany? Had Amir arranged Jaeger's move? If so, the new laboratory could be anywhere. A Saudi terrorist partnering with the German multiplied the complications: Israel could be in the crosshairs of this conspiracy. The Mossad was facing a more considerable challenge than any of them had realized.

Max called Rosh and told him, in abbreviated form, summarized everything Domenico had said. When he finished speaking, Rosh blurted out, "You have to find out where Brandt is working!"

"Rosh, along those lines, we have a bigger problem. The Swiss banker told us the Group introduced the German scientist to Amir Khan. They assigned Brandt to collaborate with the Saudi to develop more opportunities to use his lethal viruses. And we just learned from Dr. Simonson from Rambam Medical Center that Riyadh has a large, well-respected virology research facility. What if they moved Brandt's lab there?"

"We can't send a team into Saudi," Rosh said matter-of-factly. "Maybe our American allies can help us out. Do we know with confidence that they went to Riyadh?"

"We have no evidence of that," said Max. "All we know is that Khan and Brandt are collaborating, and that Brandt has abandoned his old lab."

"Assuming Brandt is not being coerced, I doubt he'd agree to go all the way to Saudi Arabia. So, if he did have to move, where would he be most comfortable moving?" asked Rosh. He offered, "Don't you think he'd try to keep the laboratory in Europe? If they're moving the lab, they need the technicians and the equipment. Max, didn't you say they left the storage freezer in the Institute?"

"Yes, a new lab would require one. We need more intel," said Max. "I'll head over to RAMOW and speak with Lev."

"Call me if you come up with something," Rosh said, then hung up.

A driver met Max at the safe house. In the car, Max called the nurse for a status report on Lilah. There were no changes in her condition, which was frustrating… but at least that meant there was no decline. Then he texted Lev to expect him at RAMOW shortly.

The brainstorming session continued at Lev's desk. Lev sipped a mug of steaming hot tea while Max caught him up to speed on the latest developments. Lev listened, wide-eyed. "If this is the same family of the terrorist killed in Colorado, then we are dealing with a shameless, bloodthirsty enemy," said Max. "They've been recruiting martyrs for years. They have resources all over the globe. Four days after the assassination in Aspen, they struck back at me in Boston."

Lev nodded and said, "We've studied the Khan family. Their M.O. over the last few years had been to blow up buses, schools, and gathering areas. This Saudi's brother was good at killing visiting Americans, like that group of Jewish athletes at the Maccabee Games in Jerusalem. And a few years ago, he bombed a soccer game played by teams with teenage Israeli and Palestinian players and killed fourteen Jewish and Muslim kids." He paused. "We thought the other brother was the ringleader, but maybe the surviving brother wanted things to appear that way. He was a few years younger, better educated...for all we know, he may have been the one directing their nefarious activities." Max nodded. Then Lev asked, "Who is their target right now—I mean, besides you?"

"That's the question," Max agreed. "They could strike anywhere, but with the Khans involved, I've got to think a Jewish target. There must be hundreds of events and conferences in Israel with Jewish foreigners and Israelis meeting every week. How many of these groups will have more than a hundred people?"

Lev typed on his computer and pointed to the results on the screen. "Here are the calendars for the state tourism bureau's activities in Jerusalem, Haifa, and Tel Aviv." There were multiple conferences every week in all three cities.

Bina piped up, "We don't know that Israel is the next target. Jews live all over the world. There are large numbers living in New York, Los Angeles, and Boston."

Max sighed, "Looks like we have our work cut out for us. We need more information. Would they strike in the United States? Or maybe this time in Europe."

CHAPTER 56

Back at Mossad headquarters, Rosh was filling Max in on the latest. "The authorities saw two Israeli Arab baggage handlers stealing packages off an airplane at Ben-Gurion yesterday morning," he said, gulping his coffee. "They couldn't catch the two guys or recover the packages. The description by the area supervisor who saw them said it was like they were waiting for those two large packages. We just learned about this now."

Max wondered whether this related to the work of Brandt and Khan. "Where did the plane arrive from?" he asked.

Rosh didn't know, but he promptly called the desk of the Mossad analyst who had taken the call from airport security. She didn't know the answer either. Rosh, incredulous, instructed her to find out immediately.

Releasing a virus in Israel is even more brazen than trying to gun down Lilah and me down a dark road in Germany, Max thought. This terrorist was consistently aggressive and way ahead of them. But who or what, beyond Max was his target? Could it be Israel?

Max called Lev at RAMOW on speaker, relayed what he had just learned from Rosh, and asked, "If the packages contain equipment capable of spreading a virus, what location do you think is likely for them to target? If he's bringing a virus to Israel, he plans to kill Jews."

Lev responded, "There are many conventions in Tel Aviv and Jerusalem, and some in Haifa. Other than the Knesset, the largest space is the Charles Bronfman Auditorium. If that's their target, then—hold on…" Lev looked something up immediately on his computer and exclaimed, "Max, the ACFI is meeting there this week! The opening session is tomorrow at noon! That would be an ideal target with Jews from around the world and many from the USA. That's got to be it!"

Rosh overheard Max's conversation with Lev and looked up. "I'll need as many agents as you can spare," Max told him. "Also, I'll borrow some from the RAMOW team to visit the ACFI Convention with me. We should go see the place today before the opening session." Max told Lev to send him blueprints of the building: the exits, layout, and structure of the HVAC system.

Overhearing Lev and Max's conversation, Bina spoke out loud, "The humidity and force of the air conditioning in that place would be ideal for spreading the virus."

Rosh said, "I'll alert the police and the security of the Bronfman Center to converge on the auditorium and get you access immediately."

Less than two hours later, Max and his team of seven met at the stairs in front of the auditorium. Despite the reluctance of the CEO of the Bronfman Center, Yitzhak Cohen, the Mossad team got into the hall, and converged in a control room at the back of the auditorium.

"Who is the manager of this facility?" asked Max. Then, from the entourage that accompanied Cohen's team inside, a voice piped up. "I am. My name is Avram Shalansky." He was a tall, broad-framed man who spoke Hebrew with a thick Russian accent. He wore a heavy belt of tools that jangled when he walked.

"Mr. Shalansky," a member of Max's team said in a strong, clear voice, "please turn the blueprints so we can orient ourselves from this room."

Avram did as he was told. In layman's terms, he described the HVAC system explaining how the air flowed inside from four outdoor vents, called economizers, situated at the four corners of the auditorium. The air was then humidified before fans dispersed it through the building via large ducts.

"If you locked the other doors," Max asked, pointing out through a control room window into the vast auditorium, "where did those people over there come from?"

"Those are not attendees. They are some late-arriving exhibitors who had entered earlier to set up their booths," said Avram. "The exhibits surround the sides and back of the auditorium."

"What are they exhibiting?" asked Max's colleague.

"A host of things. Some booths sell Judaica; some are travel companies selling trips through the Middle East. Others exhibited non-profit opportunities to invest time and money in solving issues faced by Israeli Jews and Israeli Arabs."

"I need to see a list of all the exhibitors," said Max. He and his team explored the building. Walking around inside the auditorium, they found the main shaft of one of the four intakes sealed and locked with heavy combination locks. Avram Shalansky, whom Cohen had assigned to walk around with Max, grudgingly gave Max the numbers to open the padlocks to inspect the airshafts.

"Are there any other ways to access the flow of air entering the auditorium?" Max asked.

"Well, this is the primary connection to one of the four outside sources of air. The three others are identical." The man looked increasingly annoyed. "Is this necessary?"

Staring directly into his face, from six inches away, "Yes," said Max with the sternest look imaginable. "We need to see them, now!"

"Fine. Follow me," said Avram sheepishly.

While they walked over to another location for air intake, Max said to him, "I want two security guards at this location twenty-four hours a day from now until the conference ends. You'll probably need at least two teams for each of the four shafts. Make sure we can communicate with them on our internal wireless network." Avram Shalansky did not know where he was going to find more guards.

Just then, they heard a very loud grinding and screeching sound from inside the shaft.

Looking at Shalansky, Max demanded, "What the hell was that?"

With eyes widened and his brow contracted, Avram spoke: "I don't know. It sounds like one of the major fans just broke down." He looked baffled. "I can't believe this. I'll get my crew up here ASAP and fix it. Otherwise, it is going to be an intolerably hot conference."

"I have a question," said Max. "Can you show me the outside mechanism where the air is cooled before it is sent inside?"

Staring back at Max with incredulity and a sweaty brow, "As you can see, I have a big problem. I need to be here when my crew arrives to fix this fan."

Max ordered him, "I'd prefer you to accompany us around the place. Tell one of your men to wait here for the repair crew and call you."

Max and two agents followed an indignant Avram outside. Fifty meters around the corner from the front entrance stood one of the large economizers that Avram had mentioned. Incredibly, only a simple, six-foot chain-link fence protected this vital equipment. Max thought *This is a security nightmare.*

Max instructed Avram, "Just like the four inside primary connections, we're going to need another two guards placed at each of these four outside locations around the clock." Max realized he needed at least another dozen guards, so he asked Rosh to arrange. He thought, *If only we could close the auditorium until we find Brandt and the Saudi.*

As he called Rosh to ask him to send more guards, Max realized he wasn't sure that this place was the target. It was their best bet.

CHAPTER 57

The Action Committee for Israel Convention was scheduled to begin at noon. Lev had received an update from Max's team. He sat at his desk scrolling through the list of exhibitors on the conference's website. His parents had once supported this progressive, generous, and socially responsible organization. But after Lev's childhood, the ACFI had evolved towards the opposite end of the ideological spectrum., thanks to one extraordinarily wealthy and conservative American Jew who had become the organization's primary benefactor.

As Lev studied the list, it didn't take long to recognize that several organizations seemed incongruous with ACFI's political leanings. He highlighted three on the screen. "Mac," Lev looked over at Ivan, who sat next to him, "What do you think of this?"

Pointing to the highlighted names, Lev said, "These three don't fit. They raise funds for social welfare-type projects in Gaza and the West Bank. The ACFI is so right-wing, what are the chances that anyone attending the conference would give a shekel to these guys?"

Ivan nodded, "I see what you mean, boss."

"Will you check out these organizations? Find out when they started, who started them, and where do they get their major funding."

"I'm on it." Ivan walked over to his desk.

Meanwhile, back at the Bronfman Center, people were assigned to watch the entrances and the four HVAC vents. There were two agents out front, one on either side of the glass double doors that would open at the start of the convention. Each agent operated a unique facial recognition camera on a tripod.

Max's phone suddenly rang, and he stepped outside. It was Lev calling to tell him about Ivan's discovery: all three pro-Palestinian organizations listed as exhibitors had received their initial funding from sympathetic American donors, and all three had been in operation for at least five years. But Ivan had found a fourth nonprofit exhibitor, who had been added to the convention after the initial participant list had gone to press. It was called "The Future of Palestine." The group had a minimal presence on the Internet, with only a single home page that showed that the site was still under construction. Ivan had searched for the organization's funding sources and had come up empty.

Max directed one of his team members inside the auditorium to go to the exhibitors' space and find "The Future of Palestine" booth. Twenty minutes later, the agent called him back from inside the building.

"Max, all the booths were set up yesterday, including "The Future of Palestine." It's one big Palestinian booth comprised of several groups working together at this conference. I showed the three men working at the booth the photos of the two baggage handlers. They didn't recognize them. But here's the thing: yesterday, there were five guys at this booth, and now there are only three. What if the other two guys are the ones we're looking for?"

"Get the fingerprint people over there. I want to know if our guys entered yesterday with the other three," answered Max. "And if you can postpone the start of the convention, do it!"

CHAPTER 58

After their stressful night, Rayan and Jafar slept late. It had been 2:00 a.m. by the time they'd completed the set-up and loaded the vials of cloudy liquid into the viral guns. They planned to trigger the device at noon that day when the convention was scheduled to start.

Feeling congested, Rayan awakened first. He blew his nose and saw bloody mucus in the tissues. "Jafar, I need you to wake up. I caught an awful cold," said Rayan.

Awakening with blurry vision and his eyes crusted, Jafar had difficulty clearing his throat as well. He sat up and spit bloody mucus on the floor. "I'm sorry about that," he told Rayan, embarrassed. "I can't catch my breath; my throat feels like it's closing up."

Rayan responded, "I also have a throbbing headache. How did we both catch colds?"

"I think we should just try to sleep it off," Jafar answered, coughing as he spoke. "Maybe we got sick from the guy who gave out the badges. I am going back to sleep," he coughed again, "and you should, too." Rayan and Jafar had no way of knowing that they were the most wanted men at the Bronfman Center, where the Mossad had spent the day searching for the two culprits who had stolen the packages.

Amir, sitting in an office in his Baden-Baden warehouse laboratory, was looking to hear from Rayan and Jafar, too. He had not received confirmation of the plan from them, and he was starting to get worried. Since yesterday, Amir's other friend in Tel Aviv had been reporting hourly on the plan's progress. But now, when Amir called him at the convention center, his friend reported not having seen the two accomplices since they had received their badges the day before.

Rayan and Jafar never got out of bed that day. They took turns leaning over the edge of their beds, coughing up bloody mucus, finding it harder and harder to breathe. The DVD had instructed either of them to hit the ten-digit cell phone button combination that would trigger the dispersal of the virus in the auditorium remotely, but the two men were too sick, even for that.

Amir was outraged that he hadn't heard from the two baggage handlers he had paid in advance. They had answered none of his multiple calls. By 11:45 a.m., Amir's friend told him he saw added security at the Bronfman Center's entrance. The opening of the conference was being delayed by at least thirty minutes. Amir asked himself if it was better to wait another hour before releasing the virus. Infuriated, fearing something was amiss, he impulsively punched in the ten-digit number to his phone. It triggered the devices, starting their enclosed fans, opening the valves to the chilled glass vials, and dispersing the virus into the ventilation system and throughout the auditorium.

By the time Amir entered the code, crowds had already gathered at the front entrance of the Bronfman Center. It was after noon; it was hot, and the people were getting restless. At last, the doors opened, more than an hour behind schedule. The slow line sped up once people got inside the auditorium, and everyone ran to get good seats for the opening remarks.

Ten minutes after the doors opened, Max and two agents arrived to see a long line of people waiting to get inside. They checked in with the agents operating the cameras, but they hadn't identified anyone of interest. *They must be here!* Max thought to himself. He called one of his agents inside the auditorium, only to learn that the two men were still missing.

Curiously, the agent offered, "I did notice a few men getting up from their seats coughing and heading towards the bathrooms."

Oh my God, thought Max, this *could* be it? He thought he should just empty the auditorium now, but he didn't want to create a stampede. He had to verify an attack before ending the convention and calling the hazmat team—didn't he?

He ran around outside the auditorium and encountered one of the building's security guards, apparently on a smoke break. The guard said, "I can't believe someone left their garbage collection truck there. The two guards who arrived this morning are standing next to it. I'll call the local police to get them to move the truck."

"Where?" asked Max.

Pointing to a barely noticeable back end of a truck, "Behind the auditorium," said the guard. "Over there—I'll show you."

Max followed the guard several hundred meters around to a street at the very back of the building. As he approached, Max saw the two guards standing next to a garbage truck that was obscuring the view of one of the four outdoor air intakes for the building. He felt an immediate surge of concern. "No, don't call the police," he said, "Call the hazmat team here, now."

Max ran towards the truck. He stopped in front of it and put his hand on the hood, which told him the engine was cool. It had been there a while.

Max addressed the two guards. "How long have you been here?"

"We've been here since 6:00 a.m., without a break," one guard complained.

"Was the truck here when you arrived?" asked Max, incredulous. Looking around, he saw the fenced-in outdoor economizer. The fence around the sizeable box-like structure looked to be intact. Just to make sure, he walked over to the fence and squatted down—and then he saw the gray duct tape connecting the chain links. "Cordon off this area, now," he said to the two agents who had just arrived at the site. "Get the hazmat team here, stat! We need to check this!" Even as he said it, Max had a sinking feeling that he had already missed something.

CHAPTER 59

Most of the hazardous management team arrived at the front entrance, and a contingent of four personnel met Max behind the auditorium. Like the rest of the hazmat team, they gave Max and the two other Mossad agents bright yellow hazmat suits with "HZMT" in large, red letters on the back. Finally, they donned large face masks that attached to their hoods. With a wrench, one of the Mossad agents removed the outside panel of the economizer. After climbing up into the vent, they all froze when they saw two strange-looking devices, each of which looked like a three-foot-high, tilted satellite dish covered with steel mesh. Each sheet of wire mesh sat on top of a long, twisted cone with a box at its base, and both were making a humming noise.

One look and Max knew he was too late, again. His gut contracted as if he'd been punched. On the comms system in his ear, Max called out to his team, "Close the front entrance *now*! Evacuate the building! Carefully guide the people at the entrance to move as far away as possible but avoid a stampede. The hazmat team should arrive out front. Coordinate with them." Even as he barked the orders, he berated himself. Why hadn't he had the foresight and authority to close the auditorium the moment he suspected a problem? Why had he been so sure that the virus wouldn't be released until the official start of the conference?

One member of the hazmat team drew Max's attention to the base of each of the two devices. The glass container, the size of a coffee cup, was empty. All that remained was some residual, cloudy fluid on the sides.

Shit! Thought Max.

In front of the Bronfman Auditorium, guards and agents tried to calm those running outside. There had been an announcement that canceled the convention. Everyone was asked to get up and leave in an orderly fashion, without delay. Now, everybody was scrambling for the exit as fast as they could. Many of the people leaving the auditorium were coughing, and some needed help as they felt weak and could barely walk.

The neighborhood surrounding the auditorium had become a chaotic mess. People didn't hear any explosions or see signs of a bomb, the usual cause for such excitement in Israel, but they couldn't help but react to the sirens and emergency vehicles arriving. The hazmat team had appeared and begun their work, putting up yellow tape around the outside of the auditorium and setting up a makeshift command tent twenty-five meters away from the entrance.

Dr. Hannah Feldman, the five-foot two-inch tall Director of HAZMAT Operations, barked orders into the microphone inside her special mask. With long dark hair and an athletic frame, she stood at the front of the command tent. She yelled into her phone, "This is a Code Blue Air! I repeat, a Code Blue Air! We need a full complement of support." Hearing the response, her eyes narrowed, and teeth clenched tight. Frustrated and louder, she repeated, "Yes, I said a full complement. We may well have hundreds of patients. And I need you here thirty minutes ago." Of course, she thought, *If she were a guy, those assholes would never be questioning my authority.*

Triage lines separated the people with symptoms, who were given a red flag to hang around their neck. A green one was distributed to people who had no cough, no fever, and didn't feel sick. The officers directing the process yelled out orders in Hebrew and English to segregate the conference attendees by the severity of illness. Ambulances transported the sickest directly to the hospital. Buses took those with green tags to the nursing school for observation.

It was a fact of life that Israeli disaster responders were highly experienced. Dozens of professionals and volunteers arrived and knew exactly what needed to be done. Still, as she tried to keep calm and command her team of over 150 personnel, Dr. Feldman couldn't wipe away the perspiration dripping down her face and clouding her glasses under the mask. She met with the command team of eight, who awaited her instructions. "Uri," she said to the man to her right, "update us on hospital resources."

Dr. Uri Feinberg, Director of Emergency Logistics, was ready. "As usual, Chaim Sheba Medical Center in Tel HaShomer will be our primary hospital for this disaster. The nursing school next door has been set up as an emergency field hospital. At least one hundred stretchers are there for triage." The rest of the team paid rapt attention as they heard his voice through the earbuds in their masks.

Tall and thin, in a solid stance under the puffy hazmat suit, Uri spoke with a voice that reflected his confidence and strength. He was Hannah's most dependable team member and an essential resource. She requested, "Can you update us on the potential number of victims expected?" asked Dr. Feldman.

Taking a quick scan of his notes, Uri said, "Well, the conference expected nearly 3000 attendees, including speakers and program people." He was trying to be as dispassionate as possible, although his face was sweating so much that his mask had fogged up. "In addition, there are sixty auditorium staff. Also, seventy-two booths for exhibitors were set up— but I don't know how many exhibitors were involved. I'm waiting to get those numbers."

"When you get the full list of exhibitors and attendees," said Hannah, "we have to account for everyone who walked through that entrance today."

Turning to the man on her left, she said, "Jonathan, update us on the police and IDF support."

"We have brought in every available officer in Tel Aviv," said Jonathan, a liaison from the Tel Aviv Police. "They have been assigned to manage the crowds away from the Bronfman. Two concentric perimeters were set up. The outer circle is two hundred meters from the entrance of the auditorium, with guards placed at every intersection. As a result, no one is getting in, and we are not letting people out until they have been triaged."

Hannah nodded approvingly. "Thank you, Jonathan. It's nice to depend on your department for excellent leadership in keeping everyone safe."

She turned back to Uri. "Uri, do you have any information about what is making everyone sick?" Hannah asked.

"Not yet. According to the information received so far, we are likely dealing with a potentially highly virulent flu virus, as people are getting sick fast. We just don't know how contagious it is. Therefore, we are taking maximum precautions." His cell phone dinged, and he noted a message. "Actually, Hannah, if you don't mind stepping outside for a minute, there are two people who have to see you now."

She looked at Uri, surprised at being asked to step out of her meeting. Despite being experienced in crises, Uri had never appeared as serious to her as he did at that moment. Staring at Uri, "Please excuse us for few minutes," she said to the others. "Meanwhile, contact your teams to see if they have any updated intel."

In full-body personal protective gear, Max and Lev were waiting outside the tent. Everyone was wearing masks, and yellow outfits and gloves.

"Hi Hannah, it's been too long," said Max. "Hannah was a mentor to Lilah in medical school," he said to Lev and Uri. Looking at Hannah and Uri, and I think you know Lev."

"Yes," said Lev. "Nice to see you again."

"Nice to see you Max, as well," Dr. Feldman said curtly, "but I am not sure how a cardiac surgeon can help us right now," said Hannah.

"Hannah, I am here as a Mossad agent."

Hannah's hand went to her masked forehead as her eyes widened. She paused and said, "Okay." She had changed her tune fast. "What does the Mossad have for us?"

Speaking quickly, Max shared what he had found in the economizer and what he knew about the previous viral attack in the Caribbean. Max didn't know if it would be a similar influenza virus. They had to wait and see.

"I don't know what type of virus we're dealing with," Feldman stated, "but it's different than what you found in the Caribbean. I've seen many men and some women with symptoms already. I can't believe *they* all had had HIV."

Max's shoulders tensed, and his mask fogged up more. He continued, "I'm sure you are right. I think the target population for this virus was—how should I put it?—genetically different, but specific." His furrowed brow and intense stare were obscured by the clouded mask. "Hannah, we don't want to publicize that this was a terrorist attack with an engineered virus. It's best to say it's a new flu virus that has spread, which is the truth. It will help to identify the characteristics of those infected by the virus. We need to know the age, gender, ethnicity, ancestral origin, country of origin, and sexual orientation of every person who attended the conference, not just the victims who got sick. Also, Rambam Virology Center will need specimens from everyone."

"I understand, Max," responded Dr. Feldman. "The team will scrutinize the victims once they are in the hospital. It will be more difficult for those who don't go to the hospital. I'll see what I can arrange." She was distracted by the steady flow of people stumbling out of the auditorium.

Looking into Max's face, Hannah's expression suddenly changed. "Max," she said, a hint of fear entering her voice, "people are getting sick within minutes of exposure. How are we going to stop this?"

Returning his stare through their masks, Max was silent. He said, "Hannah, we don't know. I know that you and your team will do everything humanly possible to save as many lives as possible. Thank you for that."

Hannah tried to smile. She returned with Uri to their command tent.

On their ride back to RAMOW, Max was uneasy and fidgety. Thinking of how the investigation went down, his stomach was tight as a winch, and his eyes teared. Max said to Lev, "I can't believe I let this happen. We knew about the outside condenser! We didn't have enough people watching all four intakes."

Staring at Max, Lev said, "Max, your foresight was limited by being human. You had a strong sense of what was to happen. You also had an obligation to the facts. We just weren't 100% sure. That's what we would have needed to close the auditorium and prevent this disaster."

Max nodded but felt unsettled, looking out the windows for anything to distract him.

Meanwhile, Rayan and Jafar had never made it home to Jordan. All day they had slept in their apartment. Jafar found enough strength to get himself out of bed and went to the bathroom. A spiking fever gave him the shivers. He was so weak that he had to crawl back to bed. He looked at his watch and poked Rayan, who was still sleeping.

"Rayan, wake up, wake up," yelled Jafar. "It's nearly 1:00 p.m."

The effort to open his eyes was almost too much. "What is it?" Rayan barely managed.

"We never put in the ten-digit sequence on our phones! I am doing it now," said Jafar in a panic. "I fear we failed our mission!"

Rayan responded, "I don't care. I feel so sick and am burning up with fever." He coughed up a large clot of bloody mucus all over himself and his bedsheets.

"Let's hope, praise Allah, that we were not too late," said Jafar. "I don't want to hear from the Saudi if we failed."

CHAPTER 60

Rosh diverted Max to an East Jerusalem apartment complex. Under the direction of the ranking IDF officer, Max accompanied eight soldiers, all wearing special protective hazmat gear, upstairs to the third floor of Rayan and Jafar's apartment. Both looked pitiful lying in their beds, coughing, and struggling to breathe, but Max could tell immediately that these were the two men they sought. Rayan and Jafar put up no resistance; they were handcuffed and carried out on stretchers into a windowless van. Searching the apartment, Max found the packing boxes used to ship the devices. The return address said, "Friedrich Loeffler Institute, Greifswald, Germany." He lifted the boxes and noticed that they were addressed to Rayan Jafar at the present address in East Jerusalem.

In his hazmat outfit, Max made his way to the van. He knew the potential danger of getting too close to these men, having seen the effects of the virus in St. Thomas. Despite the risk, he had to confirm that it was Amir who had given these men their instructions.

"How are you feeling?" Max asked in Arabic, each handcuffed to his stretcher.

Rayan answered immediately in Arabic, "I feel terrible. This cough in my chest is so painful, and I'm burning up." Jafar said nothing, but his face froze when Rayan responded. He tried to stop him from talking. Max, standing between the two stretchers, restrained Jafar's free arm.

"I am a doctor, and I can help you. But first, you need to tell me a few things," said Max.

"Anything," said Rayan. "Just make me better."

"Who arranged for you to get those packages from the airplane?" asked Max.

Neither responded.

Max took a different tack. "Look, I know Amir Khan was behind this attack. I just want to know where he was making the virus."

Jafar's eyes widened, "What virus?"

"The virus," Max said calmly, "that is making you sick right now and likely will kill you."

Rayan's eyes now looked like they might pop out of his head. "We know nothing about a virus," screamed Rayan, and then his yell dissolved in a fit of coughing. At last, he cleared his throat and said, "We set up those machines in the air vents and just left. We didn't know what was in it. We weren't supposed to get sick."

"Those machines shot out viruses and spread through the air vents. You contaminated yourselves with the virus, and that's why you're sick."

Now both men were staring at Max. Jafar remembered the latex gloves and masks that had been in the box and which the DVD had instructed them to wear, which they had discarded.

"How did the man notify you that the packages were on that plane?" Max pressed.

"Why should we tell you anything?" asked the Jafar, looking away. "You are just going to kill us."

"I don't have to kill you," Max said matter-of-factly. "The virus will do it if we don't treat you. The easiest thing to do is to return the two of you to your third-floor apartment to die and infect everyone around you. Or you can tell me what I want to know, and I may be able to help you."

Coughing up thick sputum and feeling sicker by the minute, Rayan spoke up. "He called us," he said through his coughs, "on a cell phone."

"When was the last time Amir called you?" asked Max.

"Why do you keep calling him Amir?" asked Jafar, as he had another coughing fit.

"Isn't that the man who paid you to do this work?" said Max.

Spitting and then clearing his throat, "We don't know any Amir," said Jafar.

And hearing that, Max called in the guards in hazmat suits to help him lift the two men and carry them out of the van.

"What are you doing?" asked Rayan.

"I am returning you to your apartment to die. Unless you cooperate, you are not going to the hospital."

A coughing fit overtook Rayan, and Jafar tried screaming but only succeeded in hacking up more sputum. At last, exhausted, Rayan said, "All right. Yes, his name is Amir. He paid us—" another series of coughing fits and taking a deep breath "— half the money before the job, and now—" he could barely get the words out, "—now that the job is completed, we'll get the rest." The guards returned them to the van handcuffed to their stretchers.

"Now that we understand one another," said Max, "where is your cell phone?"

"Our phones are in the apartment."

"Were you two born here in Israel?" Max asked.

After some hesitation, Rayan said, "We grew up in Russeifa before moving to Israel."

Jordanians, Max thought. The doctor in him could sense that the men's strength was fading. He had to get the information out of them fast. He asked, "When did you last speak to Amir?"

"We called to tell him the packages arrived on Tuesday from the first plane," said Rayan, after which he regretted saying. His coughing was worse, and his eyes bloodshot as he blazed with fever.

Max lit up, *there was another plane?* "Where is the second plane coming from?"

Jafar tried to lash out at Rayan but was restrained by a soldier. Staring at Rayan, with his HAZMAT mask in Rayan's face, "I asked you, what about the other plane?"

Coughing on cue, Rayan struggled to say, "It never arrived from Paris. It was delayed."

"Did the Paris flight also have two similar packages?" demanded Max.

Rayan managed to get out a nod, yes.

"Well," said Max, "I don't know if you will live long enough to see your family again, but you will have a better chance if you cooperate. Tell me, where did Amir have the virus produced?"

Feeling desperate, Rayan said that they didn't know exactly where but thought it was somewhere in Germany, from what they heard in the background. Max had learned that the plane had taken off from Frankfurt on a non-stop flight to Tel Aviv. Max alerted authorities about the second plane. Max wondered if *The lab manufacturing these viruses was somewhere between Frankfurt and Paris.*

From looking at the two men, Max judged that they couldn't afford to spend any more time answering questions. He told the driver to take them to the hospital.

All this time, the two men's neighbors in this neglected corner of East Jerusalem could barely tell what was happening. The area around the building had been isolated with thick yellow tape with warnings in Arabic and Hebrew: "Dangerous Contamination: Do Not Approach." Once the prisoners had gone, another hazmat team moved in and removed all property from the men's third-floor apartment. A local triage site was set up to evaluate any neighbors who felt sick.

Max had the bag with the two cell phones delivered to RAMOW. As his van sped down the highway towards the Chaim Sheba Medical Center at Tel Hashomer, the media was in a frenzy. The magnitude of the calamity drew everyone's attention. On the TV news, Israeli politicians tried to find someone to blame for the Bronfman disaster. Still, the doctors reported that a foreign visitor must have been the vector that spread it through the auditorium.

Meanwhile, Sheba Medical Center had over one hundred adult patients arriving with what looked like a severe flu. Most of them were men. Within hours of arriving at the hospital, most were coughing up thick, bloody phlegm. A dozen were already in the intensive care unit on respiratory support. The hospital feared running out of ventilators and reached out to all hospitals in Israel to borrow more.

Doctors lost no time harvesting multiple victims' sputum specimens and sent them to Rambam Hospital's virology department. As the investigation proceeded, the Center for Disease Control in Atlanta was notified. The virus samples from the Emory University attack were rushed to Israel on American Jet fighters in a flurry for comparison. At Rambam, Dr. Simonson had already received the sample from Max's surgical nurse, David Springs.

Amid all the chaos, the two Israeli Arab prisoners and three of their neighbors had been admitted to the same hospital and placed in the quarantined area. The two prisoners were still handcuffed to their bedposts. A nurse recorded in the admitting notes that these two men appeared the sickest of all the newly-admitted patients. Covered with protective gear, nurses started intravenous fluids and antiviral medications. In the ICU, they were the only men under thirty years of age requiring ventilation. It wasn't yet clear if either would survive.

As he was being driven away from Rayan and Jafar's neighborhood, Max's phone buzzed. The number on the screen was Lilah's hospital. "Hello," he answered, "this is Max Dent."

"Hello, Dr. Dent. There is someone here who wants to speak to you."

Breathless, Max thought that something happened to Lilah until he heard the voice: "Hi, sweetheart. Where are you?"

Oh my God, he thought as tears rolled down his cheeks. "It's wonderful to hear your voice!" he said, his throat tight. "I'm on my way, right now, to see you. Be there in about twenty minutes. I love you." He wiped his tears of joy.

Max arrived at the small hospital and greeted the two guards sitting on either side of her hospital room door. Finally, a nurse opened the door for Max. He was astounded to see Lilah sitting up in a chair. "You look gorgeous," Max said as he leaned over to kiss her soft lips.

An IV remained in Lilah's arm. The bandages covered the left side of her head. Except for the hair cut away from around the bullet wound, the rest of her hair was brushed back in a ponytail. She had dark patches of blood staining around both eyes, and her cheeks were puffed out. Her smile was cheerful and beautiful, despite the bruises on her swollen face.

"Now I know you're full of it," Lilah retorted. "I look like I got hit in the head with a piano! She laughed, then winced. "And it feels like that as well."

"Do you have a headache?" asked Max gently.

"A mild one," said Lilah. "The doctors said they might continue for a while. But my thoughts are clear. I don't feel any confusion. No dizziness, either."

"That's wonderful. I could use some of your insights into the challenges we are facing. But I better wait till you are ready to return to work."

"I am ready now. What do you have?" asked Lilah earnestly.

"Not so fast. We need your precious brain to recover completely," said Max as he grabbed a chair to sit face-to-face with her.

"I am so happy to see you looking so well. When did you wake up?"

Lilah looked at the nurse, who answered, "Lilah awakened around 4:00 this morning. Over the last ten hours, she got up, walked around the floor, took a shower, and ate a small meal. The doctors are very pleased with her progress." The nurse smiled. "I'll leave the two of you alone," she said, "but I'd limit your visit to fifteen minutes. Lilah still needs her sleep." She walked out and closed the door.

Max breathed a deep breath. "You are amazing. That is a rapid recovery from a concussion. I am so grateful that you are okay."

Lilah was ready to get down to business. "Seriously, Max, what's been going on? No one has told me anything, and I have no access to a TV."

How to tell her everything succinctly. "Well, briefly, earlier today there was a viral attack at the Bronfman Auditorium during the ACFI meeting. We don't have all the details, but many people got sick quickly, and too many are likely to die. We don't have enough information yet. Let's talk tomorrow after you have had a full night's sleep."

Feeling an increase in the headache, Lilah held the side of her head as she said, "Max, I am sorry for having been a burden on the mission. I feel bad you had to rush back here."

"How could you say that?" Max exclaimed. "You did everything right. They just got lucky with one of their bullets. And we got lucky. Thank God they were bad shots. But I blame myself for putting you in the situation and being unarmed. That was my tactical error." His brow furrowed as he stared intensely at her, "I never would've forgiven myself if something worse had happened to you."

Lilah shook her head gently, then suddenly grimaced as the pain surged again. "Max, thank you, but I don't remember any details. Maybe when my head clears completely, we can discuss how I ended up here."

"I know. I'll tell you everything I know tomorrow, I promise. Good night, love." Max kissed her on her lips.

On cue, the nurse returned and ushered Max out the door.

As Max walked back to the car, he tried to compartmentalize his feelings, now that he knew Lilah was on her way to recovery. He had to focus on next steps. It had been a long day already, but he returned to Mossad HQ to meet with Rosh.

CHAPTER 61

An ebullient Amir met Jaeger for lunch at Leo's Restaurant in Baden-Baden. It was one of the few places in town where Amir could eat something other than German food, which he detested. Except for the cars, he hated everything German—but today, he would put those feelings aside to celebrate his and Jaeger's shared success.

Curious, on the way to the restaurant, Jaeger had stopped at a newsstand and bought a copy of the morning paper from Frankfurt. As soon as the two sat down to lunch, Jaeger spontaneously shared his pleasure over the front-page headline: more than a hundred people had been hospitalized in Israel with what appeared to be a mysterious flu. Since the early morning, Amir had been following the international media reports of the evacuation of Tel Aviv's Bronfman Auditorium. The details were scanty, and none of the reports mentioned the two Israeli Arabs, unaffiliated with the conference, who were dying in a Tel Aviv hospital. Nor were any of the other sick Israeli Arabs described. The fact that a small East Jerusalem tenement with twenty apartments had also produced five influenza-infected patients was not mentioned, either. Based on advice from Rosh, Israel's Prime Minister emphasized in new reports, that the recent flu outbreak in Tel Aviv was just that and not a terrorist attack.

Sitting in a booth sequestered away from the other patrons, each with mugs of cold beer, "Let's celebrate our trial in Israel," Amir said as he clicked beer mugs with Jaeger, smiled, and sipped his beer. Jaeger took a long draw of chilled Paulaner Salvator Doppelbock, his favorite Bavarian beer. Before Jaeger could get a word out, Amir said, "Let's discuss our next plan. When do you think you will have enough virus to kill thousands?"

Not liking the feeling of being pushed, Jaeger responded, "Don't you think we should wait 'til we get all the data from this trial?"

"What do you need to know?" asked Amir.

"We need to know how many male and female fatalities they had. I need data to know how to scale up our next operation."

Getting a little suspicious, Amir nodded. "Don't you worry, Dr. Brandt. We'll get all the data for you." Amir decided to call his friend in Tel Aviv for more details than the news reported. "In the meantime," he said, "I thought we could talk about our next steps."

Jaeger looked up at Amir, feeling exasperated. "Okay. What do you have in mind?"

"How small can you make the viral guns?"

"I miniaturized the viral guns for my trials in Atlanta and St. Thomas. They were small enough to fit inside an aerosol air freshener. Would that size do?"

"They will need to be flatter," said Amir. "What if someone took a small virus gun and walked outside, shooting it continuously for 250 meters? Could the gun keep spraying virus the five minutes it takes to slowly walk that distance?"

"With that size of a gun, it would need a much larger reservoir," responded Jaeger.

"How big?" asked Amir.

"Probably one cubic centimeter would be plenty. Then, we'd have to aerosolize the virus by adding more saline. The virus is carried by tiny little droplets of saltwater which are propelled by forced air. Indoors, the critical factors are controlled, such as the humidity, the wind current, and the temperature. But to do this effectively outdoors, you'd have to deal with the same factors without being able to control them."

"So, we could shoot the virus walking around a large outdoor setting!" Amir responded triumphantly.

"I am not sure what you are thinking. How many guns and how much virus do you need?" asked Jaeger.

During the question, a waitress approached. Jaeger held up his hand dismissively. "Give us a moment," he ordered, not looking at her. She walked away, looking a bit miffed.

"We need enough virus to infect 200,000 people," answered Amir, "and enough guns to spray it outdoors. I estimate that you will need to manufacture 300 guns. The plan calls for a man to carry a gun and walk 250 meters and continuously spray for three to five minutes."

"That's a lot of viruses," Jaeger said, looking somewhat dubious. "And each sprayer will need a large reservoir." He paused, then asked, "Are you asking for continuous spraying over the total distance, or would you consider an on/off switch to the gun? That would make the spraying more direct and save wasted spray between people."

Liking what he was hearing, Amir's eyes lit up. "An on/off switch is brilliant. Can you design that into the guns?"

"Of course," said Jaeger with a smile. "It would be an electronic switch that is controlled by a button. How do you want to position the device?"

Amir explained in more detail how he wanted the gun and button to function. How and where he planned to use the devices would remain a secret.

"Just tell me what you need to make it happen," Amir said. "Whatever resources you require, I promise our team will provide them."

Jaeger found the plan satisfactory. He looked up and motioned for the waitress to return. "Let's toast to that," he told Amir. "And let's eat! I'm famished."

CHAPTER 62

Max had slept soundly last night, alone in their Natanya apartment. It was the first night he had rested well since Lilah's injury. This was going to be a busy day, but he got Lilah up to speed as promised. He could use her input. Max had contacted Rosh, who agreed and had arranged for Lilah to get a laptop, TV, and new cell phone for her hospital room, with access to all relevant information about the Group and regular updates from the Mossad regarding their investigations into the viral attacks.

Later that morning, when the equipment arrived, Lilah called Max. "Wow, you were serious!" she giggled. "I'll review all the notes and get up to speed." Looking at the laptop's screen, she went on, "I'll begin looking at Domenico's hard drive and the interviews. I see that I'll have access to the data coming out of Chaim Sheba Hospital as well. The early results are frightening. We've got to stop these bastards. Where do you think they moved the lab from the Institute?"

Thrilled to hear Lilah sounding as sharp as ever, Max responded, "Not sure about that. When I hear something, I'll let you know. Check-in with Lev and the team at RAMOW. They are looking into a few things." He paused. "Don't overwork yourself," he added.

"Max, I love you. I am so glad to be a part of the team," said Lilah. He could hear her smile through the phone.

Back at Mossad HQ, Rosh had prepared for an encrypted video conference with his peers at the CIA and MI5 by getting updates from Max and the RAMOW team. The virus released at the conference, he told them, might be an engineered virus like the influenza virus of 1918. Once Rosh had finished speaking, the CIA director, Gary Cummings, broke into the conversation.

"I am sorry to hear that, Rosh. Listen, this reminds me of something that happened back in December of 2012," Cummings began. "A group of virus cultures disappeared from the Rocky Mountain NIH Laboratory in Montana. At the time, I was a CIA Division Chief and heard about it from an FBI colleague. They never found the cultures, nor did they identify the thief. There was a list of foreign researchers working in the lab during a six-month fellowship. The NIH didn't want to antagonize their international partners by accusing anyone wrongly, so they dropped the case. But now I'm wondering if this has anything to do with the current situation. Let me find out who was on the list and what viruses went missing."

Rosh said, "Thank you, Gary. Yes, we need to see that list. And I believe we need to invite France and Germany into this conversation. Because of our recent misunderstandings with French intelligence, I can't call France. Gary, do you think you can reach out to them? I'll contact our colleague in Germany at the BND. They need to know what's happening. We had one attack here in Israel, and I fear we won't be the last place they strike. Let's have another call in a few days after we gather more intel."

"Shmuel, one more thing," Gary cut in, using Rosh's proper name. "You probably heard about the deaths a month ago in a hotel on St. Thomas Island in the Caribbean. An FBI colleague told me they think it was an attack of an influenza virus that specifically selected certain people and ignored the others. It was a very aggressive virus, killing everybody who got infected in just a few days. Our CDC has the updated info on the virus."

Rosh responded, "We have not yet identified the virus in the Tel Aviv attack, but yes, I learned from the CDC that they identified the modifications in the virus used in St Thomas. They also identified similar alterations in the virus that caused the death of those four college students in Atlanta this past November."

The CIA director felt embarrassed that he hadn't known about the Atlanta infections. All he could say was, "Yes, of course."

"I don't know the specifics," Rosh continued, "but we will get back to you when we learn more about the virus we're dealing with here." Rosh decided not to acknowledge that one of his agents had visited St. Thomas and had helped identify the virus at his hospital in Boston. The CIA and MI5 would never believe it was just a coincidence!

Speaking for the first time in the conversation, Inspector Clive Waller of MI5 added, "That's quite a problem you have, Shmuel. I hope the bloke stays away from our shores. I wish there were something I could do to help. Thank you for keeping us in the loop."

"Thanks, Shmuel, for the update," said Gary. "Let me know if there is anything else we can do to help."

Rosh had a favor to ask, "Gary," he began, "there is one request I'd like to make that I believe we all may find helpful."

"What did you have in mind?" asked Gary, a bit nervously.

"Well," Rosh said carefully, "the Mossad has a brilliant analyst, a psychiatrist, who has organized our database on the virus attacks. Also, she has a special interest in assessing criminal behavior. Would you include our analyst in any joint conference so that she can keep you up to date with our information, and you share with her your findings?"

Gary trusted Rosh and responded, "I'm okay with that. I plan to set up such a conference call next week. Just send me the analyst's contact info. What is his name?"

"*Her* name is Dr. Lilah Fischer, M.D., you won't be disappointed with her participation. Thank you again, Gary."

"Of course," said Gary. "We'll be in touch."

CHAPTER 63

Meanwhile, in the center of RAMOW, Max, Lev, and Bina, and Lilah—who had joined them on a video call from the hospital—stared at a spreadsheet showing a list of names and addresses of all the people admitted to the Chaim Sheba Hospital from the ACFI conference. The chaotic fallout from the tragedy had slowed the process of identifying and triaging the patients. Many of the conference-goers had not cooperated with the evacuation. Frightened, they had resisted being herded into buses by security dressed in full-body hazmat suits and helmets. Many at the hospital were getting sicker by the minute, coughing up thick sputum and feeling achy and feverish.

Sitting around the desk, Max and his team perused the list of attendees from the USA, Canada, France, Australia, and South Africa, mostly Jewish names. Bina pointed out to Max that the hospital admittees were disproportionately men, although most attendees were women. Then she noticed several with obviously non-Hebraic names and local addresses near Jerusalem. Max looked at these six Arabic names, two of which he recognized immediately. But why did the virus attack Israeli Arabs as well as Jews? "We are assuming," Max told his colleagues, "they engineered this virus to infect certain people based on their genetic identity. Now, if we work backward and understand who got infected, the targeted genetic identities should be apparent. I'd assumed the target was just Jews, but maybe not."

Lev asked, "Is it possible for this virus to be so selective?"

"Yes," said Max, who then told the group about St. Thomas and Atlanta. "Obviously, the virus released here had a broader target, since it infected some non-Jews in the auditorium. We'll wait to see what the team at Rambam finds."

Eager to share newly acquired information, Ivan had been waiting patiently to speak up. Now he said, "We followed the lead on the freezer manufacturer. For years, this French company has sold virus vaults all over the world. In the last six months, three new vaults were purchased and scheduled for delivery to Riyadh. You probably know that after our Rambam Hospital center, they have the biggest virology laboratory in the Middle East."

Max's face lit up, "Good work Mac! Find out if they took delivery on all three or if one found its way to Germany."

"I'm on it," said MacIvan.

"Lev, has your team made any progress with the two cell phones we confiscated from the two attackers?" asked Max.

"We remotely opened the phones using AI. It took three minutes for our computer to get past the passwords and found only seven numbers called by the two of them. One of those numbers on each phone was that of the other phone, of course."

"That's progress," said Max. Looking at Lilah on the screen, he said. "Lilah, maybe you can locate where the calls to our two attackers originated."

"Sure, Max," Lilah responded. "Rosh will help me with the cell phone localization. Then, once I get the region, I'll contact the satellite imaging department to identify buildings in that vicinity compatible with housing a biologic laboratory."

"That's great," said Max.

In a conference call that followed, Rambam Hospital's specialists, shared observations that surprised Max. They noted that since Jews and Palestinians lived in proximity for over a thousand years, some gene pool sharing was expected and could explain how both groups were infected.

No sooner had the virologists hung up than Max found himself face to face with an animated Ivan, "Whatcha got, Mac?" asked Max, seeing his enthusiasm.

Animated as never before, Ivan said, "We followed the lead on the freezer manufacturer. Going through their records, of the three ordered by Riyadh's lab, only two were shipped there." Ivan paused, keeping everyone in suspense. "Based on car travel times by the company's technicians we narrowed the location for delivery to either eastern France, or the western part of Germany, west of Stuttgart. Towns in that area include Karlsruhe, Baden-Baden, and Offenburg."

"Mac, share your info with Lilah who is working this from a different angle. I think the two of you may have solved our dilemma. Good work Mac!" smiled Max.

CHAPTER 64

At Rambam's virology laboratory, Dr. Shima Simonson was sitting in a conference room with two of her most experienced microbiologists. They had just completed a routine Virochip analysis, which is a pan-viral microarray platform, of two specimens: one from Chaim Sheba Hospital and the other from Max's surgical nurse, David Springs, who had died in St. Thomas.

"It's unbelievable," said the first microbiologist. "This is clearly H1N1 influenza, the same virus that killed millions one hundred years ago. But it's also different. There are a few changes in the DNA. How is that possible?"

The second scientist nodded, adding, "Someone must have altered the gene sequence! It's confusing because there are at least three varieties of the H1N1 virus in the specimens recovered from Tel Hashomer. The samples from St. Thomas contained a different type of H1N1 virus. These are previously unrecognized variants of the H1N1."

Dr. Simonson commented, "Perhaps we can figure out their significance. First, let's look at the gene sequences you have already identified. We need to know whether this virus had a specific target."

The first assistant displayed three lines of letters on the projected screen. Each set of letters represented a protein. The specific combination of the proteins, set in a particular order, determined the behavior of that virus. Next, Dr. Simonson instructed her team to run the sequences through the computer program containing the entire genome.

"Oh my God," said Dr. Simonson, recognizing the protein sequences projected up on the screen. "The sequence is specific for the Y chromosome of the Kohanes." She hadn't seen this genome for fifteen years, when her research had defined the present-day Cohens or Kohanes as true ancestors of Biblical Aaron. "I can't believe that anyone could have engineered such a feat."

Shima picked up the phone and called Max. "The good news about the virus," she told him, "is that it is not pure H1N1, which could infect anybody. In that case, we'd have an epidemic on our hands and possibly a global pandemic. Fortunately, the versions of H1N1 we isolated attack only select groups. One virus strain deployed at Bronfman was aimed at the Y chromosome of the Kohanes—you know, the group believed to have descended from Aaron. It's carried on the Y chromosome, which would explain why the virus affected primarily men."

"Fascinating," said Max. "And the other viruses?"

"We haven't decoded the others yet."

"So, you're telling me that whoever manufactured the virus was trying to kill Jewish men!" Max exclaimed. "Shima, what percentage of Jewish males have that protein sequence on their Y chromosome?"

"Max, that's a good question. Considering there has been some dilution of the genetics over the past three millennia, about fifty percent of men who claim to be Kohanes in their patrilineal origin have the identifiable Y chromosome. But I don't know the percentage of Kohanes in our general population of Jews."

Max asked, "Any thoughts on a directed treatment or a vaccine?"

"Our biomedical pharma team is looking into both challenges now. I am hoping they will have a vaccination available soon. I'll let you know when we have something."

"Thank you, Shima," said Max, as he ended the call.

CHAPTER 65

His face tight and teeth clenched, Gustav Schröder spoke into the phone: "Altman, this is Gustav."

"I was expecting your call," replied Altman Ansel. "What the fuck is going on? Is that flu outbreak in Israel Jaeger's work?"

"I don't know," answered Gustav. "It has to be Brandt and Khan. What a bold move! They struck in the heart of Israel. If it was them, I want to know what's next. I don't like surprises."

"Yes," agreed Altman. "And where the hell is Bernard?"

"He never returned to the bank or his home," responded Gustav. "My company sent four of my security guards to fetch him, and all four have disappeared. We don't know if they killed Domenico before they disappeared. I spoke to Beau, and he agrees we should meet. I'll be in touch with the date and time."

"I am very concerned," Altman agreed, but his calm voice was as unemotional as ever. "I don't understand how the guards disappeared. Something's wrong."

The next day, the three remaining Group members met in Vienna. They flew with Gustav 320 kilometers from the city's small private airport to his mountain hideaway in Obertauern on his Sikorsky S-76 helicopter.

The mountain, known for superb late spring skiing, was complemented by an azure sky view. The low altitude flight revealed the treeless slopes filled with skiers. None of the three shared any enjoyment for the vivid vistas as they waited to arrive. Nor did they see the high-altitude flight of a Starling Jet helicopter following their journey.

In the soundproof cabin of Gustav's helicopter, "This Tel Aviv attack has to be Brandt's work," growled Beau.

"I agree," said Gustav, adding with a condescending tone, "but he didn't carry out an attack of this magnitude on his own?"

"He couldn't have!" Ansel exclaimed. "That asshole had help from someone—and my money is on the Saudi."

Beau nodded. "I agree. Khan must be bankrolling the project and using his network. To think that they would go behind our backs!"

"Even if the outcome suits our purpose," said Ansel, "we can't let them get away with this."

Men in black combat gear met Gustav, Beau, and Altman and drove them in two black Mercedes SUVs to Gustav's 2,000-square-meter private mountain retreat. A woman escorted Beau and Altman inside and showed them to their rooms. The stately, Bavarian-style home, constructed of oak and larch, contrasted with the white stone foundation. Although large picture windows faced the mountains, they reflected in such a way that privacy was ensured. Nonetheless, two guards in military-style outfits and dark sunglasses stood in front of the two doors, each with a handgun on his belt and an assault rifle strapped across his chest.

Most of this was visible to the Mossad agents on board the Starling Jet helicopter, with their high-powered binoculars and high-resolution cameras. From 5,000 feet, they monitored things closely. They assessed this fortress to be secure, but not impregnable.

After dinner and several bottles of Château Margaux 2000, the remaining members of the Group sat in a quiet room with the doors closed. Sitting back in his plush chair, sipping Hennessy X.O. Cognac,

Gustav began: "I don't know what happened to Domenico or the guards sent to retrieve him… they all vanished."

Altman held his head in his hands without looking up. He cut in, "We haven't found our money. The Swiss police and Department of Detectives have turned up nothing regarding Domenico or the guards." Then, with a grim face, he looked at his two colleagues and demanded, "How could this happen to us?"

Standing up, with his arms spread out to the sides Beau joined in: "We are no longer a secret. Who could kidnap Domenico and get rid of our guards? They probably took Bernard first to get to the money. But how did they know about us?"

"We don't even know who our enemy is!" Altman exclaimed in frustration. "I think it's the Americans. It could also be the Israelis, but my bet is the Americans."

"I have a different question," Gustav cut in. Beads of sweat dripped down his face. Now speaking loudly and with more conviction, he went on, "What are we to think of the attack in Israel? Brandt must be responsible. He and the Saudi have not returned our calls. The Institute's director told us Brandt had moved his laboratory out one night and hasn't been seen since. We have to find the bastards.!"

Ansel jumped up, pointed his finger at Gustav sternly, and said strongly, "Gustav, you got us into this. What are we supposed to?"

A knock at the door was followed by a request to enter the room. A guard entered and walked up to Gustav and whispered in his ear.

"Excuse me, gentleman, I have to take a call," said Gustav.

After several minutes, Gustav returned and told Altman and Beau, "That was a call from my chief of security. At least half of the mystery is solved. The dead bodies of our four guards were found in two of our SUVs in a long-term parking lot at the airport. There was no evidence to suggest who did this!"

Before Gustav could continue, Beau stepped closer to him and yelled, "We are under attack! We need a plan.".

"Now, calm yourselves," Gustav ordered. "The three of us are okay. And we are safe here."

Altman quickly shot back, "I'm not so sure. If they could attack Israel, they could attack anywhere! Nowhere is safe."

Beau spoke next, "Our plan of action should be to wait for things to quiet down. Then we can regroup with a new plan."

"But we lost all the money in the account!" exclaimed Altman once again.

"Look," said Gustav, speaking with authority, "first things first. No one has attacked the three of us. We are not broke: only our special account is empty. I agree with Beau we should lie low and not meet for a while. Our plan is to just wait for a time and begin again."

Beau added, "And if we hear from Brandt, he will have a lot of explaining to do."

Meanwhile, the entire conversation was monitored and recorded through the ultra-sensitive microphones directed at the house from the Starling helicopter. With the help of a satellite, the transmissions were uploaded to the basement of Mossad Headquarters.

Once the guests were in bed, Gustav left the retreat and was quietly whisked away by an SUV to his private helicopter. Dov, the Mossad team leader, had sat in the cockpit of the Starling for hours, scheming. He was surprised that Gustav had left alone. *Well then*, he thought, *I guess we're in for Plan B.*

By early morning, Dov confirmed that Gustav's helicopter was resting comfortably in Vienna's private airport. He anticipated that the two remaining Group members would depart Obertauern by SUV. He gazed down and saw that one black Mercedes SUV was loading the two passengers to return to Vienna. After conferring with Rosh by phone and agents on the ground, Dov set his plan in motion.

The route from Obertauern included a drive over two mountain passes and through one unlit tunnel. The tunnel only allowed passage in one direction at a time; entry gates opened at one end while they blocked the other end. Every three minutes, after the last car exited in one direction, the traffic flow was reversed electronically by a system of lights.

From the Starling, Dov had communicated the plan to his team of three agents in two vans near the tunnel. One agent, who sat in the back seat, with his laptop accessing the Israeli satellite making a figure-eight geosynchronous orbit 21,000 miles overhead, took complete control of the tunnel's lights and the electronic entry gates. The other two agents, each driving a minivan, waited until the Group's Mercedes had crossed under the second overpass and was five minutes from entering the tunnel's north entrance. Driving through the south tunnel entrance, the Mossad agents made sure the gate closed after their vans had entered. From the north end, the black SUV carrying Beau and Altman maintained its eighty kilometer-per-hour speed as it entered the tunnel. They didn't know the gate had closed behind them.

As the tunnel curved to the right, Beau and Altman's driver suddenly saw headlights coming right at him. He swerved further to his right to avoid the oncoming vehicle, but so did the oncoming lights. The SUV struck the wall at high speed, and the airbags deployed. Before he had recovered from being punched in the face by the airbag, the driver felt a sharp needle in his neck and then blacked out. Altman and Beau, not wearing seatbelts, crashed against the hard plastic partition that separated them from the driver in the front. The older Altman Ansel's neck broke from the sudden deceleration; his last few breaths could scarcely be heard above the shouts of the Mossad agents. Beau Lancelot was struck in the head and knocked unconscious.

The Mossad agents moved quickly. One agent pushed the driver over and backed up the SUV enough to straighten it out. The two other agents pulled down the giant plastic mirror they had placed across the entire tunnel. They had borrowed the idea from an old James Bond movie, *Goldfinger*. One agent drove his van out in front of the SUV carrying three unconscious men, followed by the second Mossad-driven van. The SUV's radiator was leaking, but they didn't need to go much further. The agent, now driving the van in the rear, reached over to hit a few buttons on his laptop. The lights in the tunnel went on and the gates started functioning normally.

The whole thing took less than three minutes. Then the three-vehicle caravan continued down along the steep mountain road surrounded by a snow-covered landscape. They drove five kilometers towards Vienna, the lead driver anticipating one very sharp turn coming up. When instructed, the rear following van had stopped one kilometer back and turned across the narrow roadway blocking all following traffic. The lead van pulled ahead 100 meters and similarly turned across the road, blocking any oncoming traffic.

With Beau, Altman, and their driver in the Mercedes SUV, the agent steered the car to the edge of the steep drop with no guardrail. Only he would witness what happened next. He made sure the windows were up, opened his door, pulled the drugged driver into the driver's seat, locked all the doors, placed the van in drive, jumped out, and slammed the door. With its cargo of three passengers—two unconscious, one dead—the van rolled off the cliff and dropped another 500 meters before hitting the first of several rocky ledges. The SUV bounced off a few more before settling on the edge of another precipice. There was no life left inside.

The three agents made their way in their rented vans into Vienna, where they picked up Dov and the two pilots from the borrowed Starling Jet helicopter. The six then headed north on A5 and E50 for the four-hour ride to Prague, where the license plates on the vans were registered. When they reached a safe house on the outskirts of the city, Dov called Rosh, who was pleased to hear of their success.

Gustav was home in Vienna, waking up to a leisurely breakfast. He would not learn for several days of the car accident that had killed his friends.

CHAPTER 66

For the past week, Amir's team of eighteen Saudi virology technicians and engineers had been rushing to finish their work. They pushed hard, working sixteen-hour days, to grow viruses and build virus guns in the Baden-Baden laboratory.

Amir was thrilled with the team's success and gave them as much support as requested. Jaeger, despite his staunchest prejudices, now trusted Shazia to run the lab. Her team could reproduce the viruses without Jaeger's help—and without his knowledge.

When Amir and Shazia met privately, Shazia administered a live virus vaccine against the viruses her team would be using in the subsequent trial. The other seventeen workers would be inoculated as well. She assured Amir that he and the Prince would soon fund their own virus factory in Riyadh. Jaeger would no longer need to play any part in their operation.

Tel Hashomer Hospital
Tel Aviv, Israel

Meanwhile, Israel's sudden flu epidemic was putting an enormous strain on Chaim Sheba Medical Center's resources. The medical personnel had exhausted their supply of respirators, and they were canvassing other

Israeli hospitals for more. The victims of the virus experienced horrible deaths: choking, coughing up bloody sputum, developing pneumonia, and expiring shortly after exposure. More than half of the men admitted died within twenty-four hours, and another twenty-five percent died by week's end. Only two women died, both of whom had preexisting medical conditions. The two Israeli Arab suspects, Rayan and Jafar, also succumbed. Three of their apartment neighbors and five Israeli Arabs who had been in the ACFI Conference's exhibit space died as well.

Dr. Simonson and a geneticist colleague, plus a select group of leaders, attended a meeting organized by Dr. Judah Kassirer, the Chief Medical Officer of Tel Hashomer, to review what had happened. They were joined by Max, along with a major from the IDF.

"Thank you, everyone, for taking time out of your busy schedules to be here," Dr. Kassirer began. "I am going to turn the meeting over to Dr. Max Dent, who has led the country's response to this attack."

"As you all know," Max began, "it is absolutely critical that the information presented here remain confidential. Reports have already informed the public that a flu epidemic began in the Bronfman Auditorium." Max looked around the table at the solemnly nodding faces and turned to Dr. Simonson. "Shima, please update us on what you have so far."

"We have identified four different influenza viruses released at the Bronfman Center," Dr. Simonson said. "They all appear to have been engineered deliberately. The genetic sequences used in the modification of the viruses suggested that the targets chosen were men with Aaron's Y chromosome, Ashkenazi red-headed Jews, and Palestinians. In addition, there is one more sequence that we could not label."

The IDF major interrupted, "Dr. Simonson, I'm confused. If the viruses infected both Jews and Palestinians, it's hard for me to assume that a Saudi terrorist is the culprit. Is it even possible that the common genetic sequences are the same for the Palestinians and Ashkenazi Jews?"

Shima responded, "That's a good question. There is some overlap genetically, but the sequencing in the virus that killed the Palestinians is distinct. Whoever did this deliberately combined multiple biological weapons for this attack."

Hearing the major's comment, Max thought to himself, *Why would a Saudi deliberately try to kill Palestinians? That doesn't make sense... unless the German made the mix of viruses without telling the Saudi.* He kept his thoughts to himself.

Dr. Kassirer then updated the group on the status of the 131 people admitted to the hospital. Deaths included eighty-five men and only two women. Ten of the deceased men were Israeli Arabs. Seven men and thirty-seven women had survived so far, and none of them required respirators.

Dr. Simonson spoke again: "It occurred to me that, perversely, the scientist responsible for engineering the viruses did us a favor. It was better that the scientist modified the H1N1 virus before it was released. If he had released the unmodified form, it could have infected thousands and spread to millions. When he altered the virus to be genetically specific, the process turned off the natural ability to attack everyone. So," she concluded grimly, "at least there's that."

Dr. Simonson's statement struck Max: What if the next attack was even broader than this one? Max muttered to himself, "Let's pray that they don't do that."

"Hopefully, in time," Shima concluded, "we'll develop an antibody to treat and a vaccine to protect everyone." The meeting adjourned.

Max nodded, with a sinking feeling that time was not on their side. He could not rest until he'd found the lab that had made the virus.

CHAPTER 67

Brandt loved his spectacular laboratory in Baden-Baden. Within its walls, his dream was coming true. The freezer was filling up with freshly grown virus, which Jaeger assured Amir would kill every Jew it encountered. The eighteen Saudi technicians were now effectively on autopilot. Brandt appreciated their skills and professionalism. Although he never understood their Arabic conversations, he recognized their efficiency.

Meanwhile, Shazia assured Amir discreetly that his upgraded plan was in place; in fact, it was proceeding ahead of schedule. Furthermore, she promised him that Dr. Brandt suspected nothing.

Sitting in his lab office, Jaeger proudly informed Amir that, "We should have the 300 guns and virus ready for you in about three days. That's a lot of guns, but their small size made them easier to produce. Also, we made the vials larger, as you requested, and gave each one a wired on and off switch. Each gun can continue spraying the virus for up to forty-five minutes. Given how flat we had to make them, it's incredible we managed this."

Amir smiled as Jaeger patted himself on the back for their success. Then he cheerfully said, "Wonderful news, Jaeger! This attack will be our biggest yet. We should be able to infect and kill thousands of Jews through-out New York. The city will be brought to its knees."

Not knowing the specifics of Amir's plan made Jaeger uncomfort-able. But Amir had been generous, and Jaeger couldn't help but smile at the prospect of wiping out many of New York's Jews. "Yes, I am sure it will be a great success," Jaeger said.

Brandt was right to suspect Amir of lacking transparency. Thanks to their work under Jaeger, Shazia and her team had learned how to increase infectivity and lethality. As a bonus, besides the vaccines they developed to bring home, they took samples of the original H1N1 and several other viruses Brandt had hidden. Once the lab had completed production of the elements Amir needed for this attack, his skilled group of research-ers would return to Riyadh with the knowledge necessary to bioengineer genetically specific viruses on their own.

Amir, meanwhile, had arranged for the packaging of the guns and virus. The virus would ship in self-contained cooling units, labeled as Frozen Preserved Human Blood Products under the auspices of the German Navy. This would get the packages through U.S. customs. He had all the correct forms and boxes supplied by a loyal follower who had recently pilfered them. They dyed all 300 vials of the virus red so that they would resemble blood specimens.

The Saudi team dismantled the guns into three separate segments and packed them to be shipped in boxes of ten. This made them uniden-tifiable, and Amir was confident they would go unrecognized by U.S. Customs. Later that day, the gun sections would be picked up by Federal Express, and the vials would go out the next day, April 1. All the packages would arrive overnight at selected warehouses.

Amir's entry into the U.S. was another issue. He had to be there to supervise the last details—and he had to observe at least one attack. What a waste it would be if he couldn't revel in the fruits of his labors!

Initially, he considered using the Prince's jet and taking the same route through Canada by which Asif had arrived for the ski trip. But the

Prince, worried that the FBI might be looking out for the jet because of the disappearance of Asif's body, didn't want it used again outside the region. Amir realized he might have to get creative. He contacted an old friend in Argentina and arranged an itinerary to get to the U.S. by other means. At last, after reviewing a few details with Shazia, Amir left for Orly Airport in Paris.

After readying all the packages for shipment, seventeen Saudi scientists quietly returned to Paris for flights to Riyadh. They traveled in groups of two or three and used different airlines to go home to Saudi Arabia. Two guards stayed behind to help Shazia fulfill her brother's orders: destroy the lab and then take care of Brandt.

CHAPTER 68

CIA Director Gary Cummings was very concerned. "Thank you for meeting with me today," he said brusquely to his audience as his strong hands gripped the edge of the conference table. "Let me introduce everyone. To my right is senior agency analyst Dr. Arlene Robbins. On her right is Director David Wright of the FBI, and then next to him is FBI agent Thomas J. Smith, the Special Agent in Charge of the Middle East Desk. In addition, on a video conference call from Israel is Dr. Lilah Fischer, a psychiatrist, and analyst for the Israeli intelligence agency."

"Dr. Fischer," Cummings directed his gaze to the computer screen, "Thank you for being here. We want to update everyone on the three viral attacks around the globe." He turned to his right. "Arlene, would you begin, please?" Dr. Robbins described the viral outbreaks in Atlanta and St. Thomas, with a timeline projected on the eighty-inch screen behind her.

Cummings asked Lilah to do the same for Israel. After summarizing the facts, she continued, "A specialist at the Rambam Medical Center here in Israel believes that the viruses we have seen are variants of the original H1N1 influenza — the flu. You probably know that the original flu virus killed over 40 million people worldwide in 1918."

Arlene continued, "Dr. Fischer, have you established how contagious this new virus is?"

Lilah responded, "Dr. Shima Simonson, Rambam's Chief of Virology, noted that the virus only infected genetically targeted individuals. The only secondary spread of the virus was to people with similar genetics."

Feeling anxious, Director Cummings spoke, "Until the facts are clear, it seems obvious to me that travel for Americans into Israel has to stop immediately. Also, our borders should be closed to anyone coming from the Middle East."

David Wright responded, "That's not so easy to accomplish, despite its obvious potential benefits. Canceling U.S. flights to Israel is a political football. As you know, this President often decides in a vacuum, in ways that disregard science. Since he promised to make peace in the Middle East, he'll refuse any suggestion that portrays Israel in a less than favorable light—even if that decision is in the best interest of the American people."

Uncomfortable with FBI Director Wright's political concerns, Gary responded, "I wonder if the PR people can frame the recommendation that we limit travel to and from Israel until they can assure safety."

"Excuse me, may I add something?" asked Lilah.

"Sure, Dr. Fischer," Gary said, "of course."

"Thank you, sir—and please, call me Lilah. Dr. Simonson observed that viruses only attacked people with specific genetic identities. No one caught the virus from another infected patient unless they had a similar genetic identity. So, this means that for a while, until all the infected victims have been evaluated and quarantined for two weeks, it is not safe for the rest of the Israelis or foreign visitors with a similar genetic identity to visit here. Since segregating everyone by their genetics is impractical, a temporary travel ban makes sense. We'll know much more about this in the next week."

"Thank you, Lilah. We appreciate your insights," said Gary. He continued, "I think the PR people can spin this satisfactorily. Perhaps the President can acknowledge how great a job the Israeli healthcare has done to contain the virus such that the Israelis are continuing about their everyday life, just temporarily avoiding that small area in Tel Aviv."

"Fair enough," said Director Wright. "I'll send this up the ladder to the White House PR people. That should work."

Special Agent Thomas Smith, known as Smitty, jumped in, and asked, "Can the Israelis tell us if there is a relationship between the assassin's work in Aspen and the attack in Israel?"

With raised eyebrows and tight lips, Cummings looked sternly at Agent Smith and said, "That question is out of line and does not bring relevant data to our discussion to understand these attacks."

Agent Smith sat down and put his head down, knowing he had had his hand slapped.

Smitty's question had made Lilah's heart race. Her headache returned, and she felt her body tightening up. Immediately, she turned away from the camera. Did they know of her relationship with the assassin? What was she obligated to tell them?

Cummings continued, "Lilah, your director informed me you might add more insights into understanding the terrorists."

"We know," Lilah continued, trying to speak through her headache, "that the three attacks, Atlanta, St. Thomas, and Tel Aviv, resulted from an aerosolized virus that genetically selected certain populations for attack. In each instance, the victims all had genetic markers in common. Specifically, the virus struck four Atlanta college students with sickle cell trait. Seven men in St. Thomas who had had HIV years earlier died in the second attack."

Lilah then told them what she had learned from Dr. Simonson about the multiple viruses recovered from the attack in Tel Aviv. She continued, "Let me say, categorically, that everything these nefarious scientists have done in manufacturing the viruses in the three attacks has been very deliberate."

Gary Cummings interjected, "Scientists? Do you think there is more than one?"

"I don't know how many scientists it takes to engineer a virus. But to grow the virus, build the viral guns to spread the virus, and then deliver the viral guns to the location for dispersal—that is the work of at least two people, and likely more."

"Considering your expertise, what can you tell us about the likely killers?" asked Director Cummings.

"There are at least two. These individuals are aggressive," she said, and then images of the gunshots in the car ride in Germany flashed through her mind and made her falter. "…I am sorry," she stammered, "I just got a migraine." She looked away from the camera. "Give me a moment." The assembled group watched Lilah clench her teeth and then reach for a glass of water and sip it. "I am sorry," she repeated.

Dr. Robbins asked, "Lilah, are you okay to continue?"

"Yes, thank you," said Lilah, clearing her thoughts. "I'd like to summarize by saying that these murderers are ruthless, bloodthirsty, and have no regard for human life. We believe the first two attacks were 'clinical trials.' The attack in Israel was intended twice as large, as we found a second plane that arrived the next day with two more loaded large viral guns. I fear that there will be bigger attacks unless our intelligence services collaborate to prevent them."

Cummings looked grim. "Your report is sobering. Thank you, Lilah, for joining us today." He started to end the conference, but then Director Wright interrupted.

"I am sorry you are not feeling well, Dr. Fischer, but I have to ask you one more thing. Do you have any information about who the likely perpetrators are and what they plan to do next?"

Lilah answered, "We uncovered a likely collaboration between a German scientist, capable of modifying the virus, and a Saudi terrorist organization. We don't know to what extent they are working together. One more thing we believe is that the terrorist killed in Colorado is the brother of the terrorist collaborating with the German scientist."

At this, Wright jumped up and screamed at the monitor. "How come Israel has kept this so damn quiet!" Everyone stared at Wright's menacing face. Looking back at Director Cummings, "I told you so," Wright said.

Keeping her cool, Lilah replied, "The knowledge I just shared has only been verified in the last six hours. I think Director Gurion asked me to participate so the Mossad could provide you with up-to-date information. We are all on the same side in this."

Cummings, Robbins, and the others seemed to be used to Wright's outbursts. Arlene Robbins commented, "Lilah, thank you for sharing this valuable information. The fact that a Saudi is involved completely changes how we analyze the situation."

"I agree, Dr. Robbins," said Lilah. "We believe the viral designs were deliberate. What we can't explain is why a Saudi terrorist would want to kill fellow Muslims? What we do know is that this Saudi terrorist organization has sworn to kill more innocent people to bring attention to their plight. If these criminals," Lilah continued slowly, "wanted to make a bigger splash on the world stage, we must consider something on the scale of 911 or even larger."

This brought another hush to the group. Dr. Robbins piped up, "That's exactly where I thought you were going. The next attack may well be here in the U.S. or a major European city."

As Director Cummings gathered his thoughts, he murmured, "What I don't get is, what group would they select to kill on a larger scale in the U.S.?"

"Well, sir," Lilah answered, "with all due respect…let me paraphrase Dr. Simonson once again. She said that the scientist had done us a favor by selecting a small portion of the population. If he had released the unadulterated H1N1 and increased its lethality, he could have caused another global pandemic. My fear, sir, is that if they attack America or Europe, it will be with a more lethal form of pure H1N1, one without genetic specificity, and we will see tens of millions die because their old flu vaccines won't protect them."

"That sounds crazy to me," Director Wright protested. Then he added, "Does the Mossad know where the German scientist and the Saudi are at present?"

Carefully considering her response, Lilah responded, "We know the collaboration began at the Friedrich-Loeffler Institute in Germany. But they left there over a week ago. We are looking for them now. But I have made a few observations reviewing the history of this Saudi family of terrorists."

"Go on," Gary prompted.

"I would expect the Saudi terrorist," Lilah said thoughtfully, "to be present during the attack. He has a reputation for witnessing and filming many of the attacks his brother delivered. The terrorist is the Minister for Economics in Saudi Arabia, Amir ibn Khan. If you can find him quickly enough, we may be able to prevent the attacks."

"What about the German?" asked Director Wright. "Do you have more information on him?"

"We think his name is Dr. Jaeger Brandt, a geneticist. But we have no updated info on him," said Lilah. "If we uncover anything, we'll share it with you."

Director Cummings spoke, "I'll have to send this to the White House to see if I can get them to reach out to the King of Saudi Arabia. I doubt the King will be happy to hear about his Minister for Economics."

"Unless he's in on it," Wright muttered.

Cummings shot him a hard look and continued. "Lilah, you have given us a lot of information, some that we have to act on immediately. Director Wright and I can meet and plan a strategy. Dr. Fischer, if we can be of help, please let us know."

"Thank you, Director Cummings. I'll tell Director Gurion of your support. I am sure he will be in touch."

CHAPTER 69

Sitting in his office in FBI Headquarters in Washington, D.C., Agent Smith made a call. "Wally, this is Smitty. I have been trying to reach you."

Walid Manzur answered on his mobile phone while driving. "Hi Smitty," he said, "I've been chasing down some perps who stole guns from a sporting goods store in Denver. I haven't been in my office much."

"I have some follow-up for you on the case they instructed us to drop," said Smith carefully, at which Agent Manzur pulled his car over to the side of the road and to pay full attention. Smitty continued, "Well, it turns out that the family of the dead terrorist has been behind massive viral attacks around the world. The guy's brother may head here—and my sources think it's likely he's bringing the next attack with him."

"Smitty, that's terrible!" exclaimed Agent Manzur. "Is it related to the assassination of the Saudi in Aspen?"

"I knew you would ask me that. It's not a cause-and-effect thing, I don't think, but it's obviously related, in the sense that these guys were brothers and had the same extremist agenda."

"Brothers?!" Walid grimaced and clutched his steering wheel tightly as he attempted to control his anger. "I guess I should say thanks," he managed, "for keeping me in the loop that I am not supposed to be in."

There was a pause on the line. Then: "Wally, I have a question that you might be able to answer. I know you researched this Boston surgeon. Do you remember the name of his girlfriend? I remember you said she was a psychologist or something like that."

"I don't recall the name now, but it's in my files. When I get back to the office, I'll email you the name. Why are you asking?"

"Something came up, and I wanted to clarify a few things. Thanks for picking up."

"Yeah," said Walid Manzur, "Take care." After he ended the call, pangs of frustration shot through him, making him clutch the steering wheel even harder. He appreciated his career too much to risk losing it for one bad guy. But he had already put so much effort into this case! Now, he'd be damned if he didn't find that doctor.

CHAPTER 70

In the twilight hours on Sunday, a jet registered as a cargo transport landed on a private airfield not far from the Frankfurt airport, carrying Max, Ivan, and Zalman. The plane carried three electric motorcycles for transportation. They had 175 kilometers to cover to reach the likely location of the laboratory. The jet refueled and then pulled into an empty hangar to stay hidden until it was needed.

In his mind, Max ticked off the major towns as he drove south: Weiterstadt, Bensheim, Weinheim. He saw a sign for Birkenau. He knew the Auschwitz II-Birkenau death camp was in Brzezinka, Poland, hundreds of miles away, yet the name triggered his compassion for all the victims who had had no chance to survive the Nazi regime. Max couldn't save them any more than he could have saved his murdered family members—but he recalled the conversation with Aunt Gila and vowed to continue the fight.

The cloud cover and moonless predawn morning made using the GPS essential. They all stopped at Ivan's signal. "Lilah connected me with a friend in Aman, (Israeli Military Intelligence), in Unit 81, the secret technology guys. They have the best satellite intel." Max smiled at MacIvan's infectious enthusiasm. "They probably collaborated with America's NGA, I'm not supposed to know that, but they produced some critical geospatial images." Pulling a small iPad out of his backpack, he displayed a series of screens, "Between the identified cell towers, they found buildings large enough to fit the lab. But this one had activity," Ivan continued, pointing to the image, "See those trucks lining up to deliver goods here. I believe the lab is in that building."

Max asked, "Mac, why are you so confident that's the building?"

Ivan's face brightened up, as he knew Max hadn't seen all the data, "The timestamp for those images perfectly matches three days before you went to the Institute."

His eyes rolling, Max asked, "Wait, you mean we just happened to have satellites over the area before we even questioned the lab's new location?"

"No. There are hundreds of satellites circling the globe all the time. I'm told that our satellites borrowed the imagery from two satellites that were geostationary over the French-German border; one French, the other American."

Studying the images, Max smiled at their precision. First, he could see men lifting boxes and bringing them into the building, then an eighteen-wheeler deliver a very large crate. "Mac, what do you think this is?" he pointed.

"That's their freezer. Look at the markings on the truck, *Le Groupe Scientifique*. That's the name of the French freezer manufacturer!" Ivan said with satisfaction.

"Wow," was all Max could say.

They rode their quiet electric motorcycles another two kilometers down a darkened road when they reached the edge of the forest. Two large stone warehouses were in the distance, lit with corner lot lights.

They parked their cycles behind the trees and walked to the two identical buildings.

"Mac," asked Max, "which is it?"

"It's the second one," MacIvan replied. The agents went behind the building and found an opaque window on the rear side. There was a loading dock in the back, with discarded liquid nitrogen tanks strewn around the ground. To the side of the parking lot was a dark green BMW 7 Series sedan with German plates.

"This is the place," Max said. "Those cylinders on the ground once contained liquid nitrogen, which they must've used to cool the viruses for transport. We have to get inside."

Concerned, Zalman said, "I am surprised there is no guard here."

Max, noting his concerns, "You're right…not sure what that means."

MacIvan checked for infrared signals and for Wi-Fi inside, which might communicate with an alarm system. Finding neither, MacIvan said, "The loading door is tough to break through." Pointing to the side of the building, Ivan continued, "Let's knock out that window."

They cut out the window and Zalman, who was the smallest, climbed inside. He went around to the front door, opened it, and no alarms went off. They double-checked and found no security cameras.

Max and Ivan walked slowly through the space. Zalman stood inside the front entrance as the lookout. There was something ghostly about the place. The hot area where the scientists had stored viruses was evident, but the doors stood ajar. Max put on one of the positive-pressure suits just in case the BSL-4 was booby-trapped. He went inside and saw that the six freezer doors were left open and turned off. It was empty. *Shit,* he thought. *Too late again! That's why there was no guard outside.* He walked into another laboratory room with dozens of destroyed fume hoods along the counters. It was a mess, with broken glass test tubes and pipettes around the bench and littered over the floor.

"This lab was much bigger than the one in the Institute," Max said to the others. "If Brandt was manufacturing virus here, he could have produced a ton more than before."

Suddenly, Ivan blurted out, "Hear that? That screeching?" As soon as he said it, they all heard the muffled scream of a trapped or frantic animal.

"I think it's coming from over there," Max pointed to a back closet." Max gestured to MacIvan, and the two walked around with their nine-millimeter Masada pistols extended out in front until they identified where the noise was the loudest. Then, holding his gun aimed at the door, MacIvan unlocked the door to find a frightening sight. Sitting in his excrement was a naked man with his arms and legs tied behind him. Someone had cut away most of the skin on his arms, legs, chest, and abdomen.

To Max, it looked like someone used a surgical dermatome all over the man to donate skin for a burn victim. All the body's surfaces were oozing blood. Despite his years of surgical experience, Max shuddered to look at the horrible sight. Hearing the cries louder from the closet, Zalman left his post at the front door to see what they found. Zalman's hand flew to his stomach as he doubled over and retched. He turned away and tried to pull himself together.

With nitrile gloves on, Max and MacIvan reached into the closet and gently lifted the man out of the closet and onto a workbench. They cut the ropes that restrained his arms and legs, and a hideous scream escaped his mouth. Zalman walked around until he found a first aid kit. After gently washing the man off with tissues soaked in cool water, Max found clean cotton sheets from another room and covered the man's body. To Max, this skinned man's injuries amounted to a near-total body burn. Zalman started speaking to the man. Hysterical and exhausted, the man kept repeating the exact thing over and over and moaning loudly.

Zalman, in German, asked his name. The man became quiet, then he cried. When the sobbing stopped, he stared at them and kept repeating the same phrase to Zalman.

"He said, we look like Jews."

Max responded, "I know what he said. We found our man."

"Holy shit!" exclaimed Ivan. "This is the crazy scientist!"

Zalman stayed with the man while Ivan and Max walked around the space, looking for cameras that might be recording their visit. They found nothing of interest until they both ended up at a locked door. Unable to pick the lock, MacIvan had to place a small explosive to blow the door open. The smoke cleared, and they burst through the door and discovered a pile of weapons: rocket launchers, sub-machine guns, AK 47's, and enough ammunition for a small army.

They walked away from the stash of weapons and walked back towards the loading dock, where they found piles of unused, folded Federal Express boxes left on the floor against the wall.

Max tried to put this all together. This was clearly the laboratory they were looking for—but what was the deal with the FedEx boxes? Had they shipped the virus somewhere already? And where to? And what was the extensive collection of military-grade weapons for?

Ivan and Max headed back to the room where Zalman stood next to the German. Ivan avoided looking at the man. Even when looking away, Max found the sight of the man's flayed body seared into his memory. Max lifted the man's head and took a closer look. In German, he said, "Hello, Dr. Brandt." The man didn't speak, but his eyes exploded open, and his face lit up. His fear was evident, for they knew who he was.

Zalman continued, "How long have you been in this closet?"

Brandt stared away from his questioner, then mumbled, "Since last night."

"Okay, guys, let's go," said Max. "We can't just leave him here. After all, he may be of value to us."

"Will he even survive like this?" Zalman asked, incredulous.

"I'm not sure he will," said Max. "Whoever cut off this much skin left him to die an excruciating death. We can try to resuscitate him on the airplane if he makes it that far. Let's wrap him snugly in these cotton packing sheets and tie him to the back of one of the cycles."

Despite a constant flow of epithets and curse words from their frightened, pain-stricken passenger, they notified the pilots and made it to the airfield. Inside the hangar, the jet had just started its engines. The three men drove the cycles up to the cargo door and put all three inside. Then they lifted Jaeger inside, trying not to cringe at his agonized cries. The pilots were aghast when they saw the man swaddled in blood-stained wraps.

The plane taxied out of the hangar and immediately raced down the runway. Max and Zalman had already started working on Brandt's wounds. After cleansing the wounds with warm saline, Zalman covered the victim's arms and legs with Silvadene to soothe the pain and prevent infection. Max started an IV and loaded the victim with fluids, antibiotics, and enough morphine to cut the intense pain. The German saw what they were doing and couldn't believe it: these Jews were treating him better than the Arabs had. He drifted into a drugged sleep.

"We'll debrief him when he awakens," Max said. "If he survives, we'll have an ambulance waiting for him. Can't transfuse him 'til we get to Israel and check his blood type." Max shook his head. "The thought of wasting one drop of Jewish blood on this murderer kills me," he told them, "but it's the right thing to do. We may learn about the next attack. Hopefully, he is worth more to us alive."

After a few silent minutes, Zalman said, "We were late again. They had abandoned their laboratory." He sighed in frustration.

Opening his laptop, Ivan asked, "Max, what do you think about the FedEx boxes?" He connected his laptop to the satellite. "I'm going to hack the Federal Express IT system to see if they sent any packages from that address."

After thirty minutes, MacIvan got a long download of over 900 shipments from the warehouse. Some shipped two days before, the rest the next day. "Holy shit," said MacIvan. "They shipped almost a thousand packages to the United States. But, unfortunately, I can only find the destination country and no more details."

Max grimaced. The problem was even more significant than he had feared. If those packages contained devices to spread viruses, then he had to find out where they were being sent. From the plane, Max called Rosh and spent an hour debating with him about what to do next. Max proposed a plan that would require Rosh to contact the CIA first, but also the U.K.'s MI-6. He also wanted Rosh to reach out to the German BPOL and the

French DGSI about the viral attacks and the location of the weapons stash in Baden-Baden.

"Any coordinated counter-terrorism strike would be complicated, risky, and expensive," Rosh exclaimed. A moment of silence passed as Max heard Rosh's deep breath. Rosh continued, "You better be right about this."

"I am," Max assured him. "And now we know that all the packages are going to the U. S. We need to find the addresses where the packages are headed."

"What's next on your end?" asked Rosh.

A nap, Max thought wistfully, knowing it was a dream. He answered, "I'm going to call a friend at the CIA."

CHAPTER 71

O ver the last forty-eight hours, Amir had flown from Paris to Buenos Aires to Havana. But none of his jetlag or stiffness could rival the discomfort of the most dreaded leg of his journey. Amir had been seasick and vomiting for most of the ten hours he had spent on the slow fishing trawler from Cuba. He hated boats. An expensive yacht pulled up alongside the old trawler. In international waters, twelve miles northeast of Cuba, two fishermen carried the dizzy Amir off the boat and into the sleek vessel's stateroom. They gave him medications and intravenous fluids to relieve his nausea. Amir's new ride pulled away quickly and ran northeast for another fifteen miles before heading into Key Biscayne Bay, just south of Miami. The captain prayed to Allah that he would avoid the U.S. Coast Guard. As he approached the shoreline, he looked forward to discharging his nauseous passenger.

They passed into the Biscayne Bay and then northwest towards Coconut Grove. Once close enough to the mainland to see the docks, the captain felt safer. He called ahead to ask where to tie up. There were many powerboats in the inner harbor, so hiding among them was the best plan. Amir's legs were unsteady as the crew carried him into the waiting arms of two Middle Eastern men.

Once Amir had disembarked, the yacht pulled away immediately, reversed direction, and headed back out through the harbor and into the ocean. As the captain and crew headed south out of the bay, not three miles away, the U.S. Coast Guard stopped them. They had no choice but to welcome the officers on board and comply with their request to see everyone's identification. The officer then pulled out a photograph of Amir.

"Have you seen this man?" the officer asked.

Both captain and crew denied seeing him. They insisted there was no one else on board. The Coast Guard meticulously searched their boat and found nothing. The captain breathed a sigh of relief. Praise Allah, he thought, grateful that the Coast Guard had been too late.

The two loyal Wahhabis who met Amir on the dock rapidly transported him to a small home in Coconut Grove. He spent two hours there resting and freshening up. He felt more like himself now but depleted. *I hate the sea.* Amir kept thinking, even as he opened the brown leather bag that had been left for him on the dresser. Inside were 5,000 American dollars, a Florida driver's license with his photo and Malik El-Khoury's name and matching credit cards. He also found three new burner phones in their original blister packs and a nine-millimeter Beretta with 100 rounds.

The plan called for Amir to begin in Miami and meet with the loyal followers eagerly awaiting his arrival. A driver took him to the warehouse in Little Havana, three blocks from Marlins Park. The followers greeted him like a celebrity, with eighty men and women bowing as he entered the garage entrance. The door closed immediately.

Amir noticed the opened Federal Express boxes piled up along one wall.

Hamid, who believed that his visitor's name was Malik El-Khoury, greeted Amir and welcomed him. "I trust your travel went smoothly, sir," he said. Amir nodded; he wouldn't disclose his weakness for the sea. "We received the second set of boxes this morning, as you instructed."

"Allah has delivered me as planned. How are the preparations going?" Amir asked.

"Very well, sir," responded Hamid. "Allow me to show you what we have done."

In the center of the space stood seven foldable tables, each six feet long by three feet wide. On each table, the viral guns sat in various phases of assembly. Refrigerated units, cooling the virus reservoirs, sat on two of the tables, plugged into electric outlets. Amir scrutinized everything carefully.

Picking up one gun and pointing to the coupling where the two critical elements connected, he said, indicating, "You must close these fittings tightly, or there will be a leak." He looked at the little devices on all the tables carefully. Then he turned to Hamid again, "Please demonstrate how you attach these gadgets to the trays."

Hamid picked up a tray from the stack on the other side of the tables. It was a large, aluminum concession tray that vendors carry around a stadium when hawking popcorn and soft drinks to fans. This one was covered with Miami Marlins logos. He turned it upside down and attached an assembled virus gun to the underside of the tray with Velcro strips. The button that opened and closed the gun's valve was placed adjacent to the spot where the popcorn vendor—one of Hamid's volunteers—would hold on to the tray with the right hand. While each volunteer carried a tray with a strap around their necks, their right index finger could press the button on the hidden gun, releasing the virus.

Amir beamed. This was just as he had envisioned! There were seventy martyrs ready to spread the virus at Amir's command. "All of you," he addressed the group, "have made Allah proud. I will leave you now. You have two days to complete the preparation. You know," looking directly at Hamid, "how to attach the vials as we said in the videos?"

"Yes, of course, sir," said Hamid, "just as you instructed."

"And remember, the vials are not to be opened by anyone until the day our people go to work, our opening day. Do not press the buttons until you arrive on-site and begin selling the popcorn."

"Yes, sir," Hamid said. "May I have a word with you alone, please?" They walked into a back office with an opaque glass window. After closing the door, Hamid began, "We are grateful for the opportunity to serve Allah. But tell me, what does this little gadget spray as our men and women walk around?" Immediately Hamid felt the pain of Amir's intense eyes.

"The spray is harmless to our people," Amir lied. "It contains a virus—a special mixture that only attacks Jews and non-believers."

If Hamid had any doubts, he banished them under Amir's focused stare. "I understand. Thank you, sir. We will spread Allah's word as we spray the mixture."

"One more thing, Hamid: give me your mobile phone."

Hamid assented. Amir took the phone and punched in his burner's number. "You now have my phone number. In an emergency or last-minute question, you can reach me."

"*As-salamu alaykum*," Hamid said.

"*Wa'alaykumu s-salam*," Amir replied. They shook hands, and he left the warehouse. A driver took him to a small private airstrip, whence another loyal follower would fly him the 1100 miles in a Beechcraft Bonanza single-prop plane to Teterboro Airport in North Jersey.

After one stop for refueling, the five-hour fight, aided by a strong tailwind, brought Amir closer to his next location. Headphones quieted the noisy but comfortable flight. He dozed on and off until the vista of the New York City skyline filled his window. As the plane approached northern New Jersey, all Amir could think about was a good night's sleep.

CHAPTER 72

After having met with Rosh at Mossad HQ, Max stepped into a quiet office space to make a call. "Lilah, I assume you are back in our apartment?"

"It was tricky getting here," Lilah responded, "without letting the driver know where we're living. I just had my parents drop me off. They were good about it."

"Smart idea." Max thought to himself, grimly, now that she had brought her phone and laptop into the apartment, Rosh could find their location.

Having heard about the night trip to Germany, Lilah was thrilled to hear Max's voice. She shared his frustration in trying to stop another attack. Attempting to be upbeat, Lilah said lovingly, "You've been a busy guy."

"Yeah, well, we found the German scientist, or what's left of him. He will need skin grafts over eighty percent of his body, blood transfusions, and metabolic support for the next three weeks if he is going to live. The value of keeping him alive is to learn as much science from him as we can. Maybe he can tell us about the next attacks. After that, I don't care what happens to him."

"I am sure they have plenty of German speakers, so they won't need me."

"Lilah, I am grateful for your willingness to help," said Max, "but you have done plenty already! I heard from Rosh that you told the Americans you think the Saudi will want to witness the attack. That was perfect! If nothing else, that may get them to help us find him. Also, they won't be shocked when we show up there tomorrow."

"Max be careful," said Lilah. "We don't know what kind of virus they plan to release this time—and we don't know how they are going to do it." She paused. "I love you."

"I love you, too. Don't worry," he added. "I'll see you in a few days."

CHAPTER 73

After Amir finished breakfast at a small hotel in the Bronx, a short, thin, swarthy man greeted him out front. His clothes were modest but clean and well-fitting.

"*As-salamu alaykum*," the driver said to Amir. Seeing the heavy leather bag Amir had in his right hand, he reached out and asked, "May I carry your bag for you, sir?"

"No, thank you. I am fine." Not fully rested and feeling anxious about being in New York, Amir needed to maintain an air of superiority. As they walked through the poorest congressional district in the United States, he could see the dramatic disparities between the haves and have-nots. There were luxurious, affluent homes with small grass plots in front and on the sides, surrounded by six-foot-tall black steel fences. Just four long blocks away stood impoverished tenements. While walking through neighborhoods, Amir knew, of course, why his fellow Wahhabis had settled in this densely populated area: they had sought a community of fellow Muslims. The forty-two square miles of the Bronx housed a significant Muslim population. 20,000 Wahhabis prayed at the largest mosque in the district. They were educated but lived simply. Amir had chosen this non-violent community as his point of contact for this operation, sure the local Muslims would welcome a member of the faith.

After a few blocks of silence, Amir looked at the man, "Where do you live?"

Surprised Amir had asked, the man pointed behind them and answered, "Two streets over, in the opposite direction."

"Do you enjoy your life here in New York?"

Considering how best to answer this highly respected man from Saudi Arabia, he said, "I like my life here. Both my wife and I work, and our children are educated at the mosque."

Curious, Amir asked, "What does your wife do?"

"She is an excellent seamstress. She repairs and makes dresses for an expensive dress shop in Manhattan. They pay her very well," the bearded man answered proudly.

Amir responded, "That is good. I am happy for you." Amir, in a moment of warmth, studied the unassuming man before him: a family man, a good Muslim. Hopefully, the virus would not strike him.

Amir observed the covered women walking on the streets as he passed by. They never walked alone, always accompanied by their husbands or by several other women. This community would understand the need for his attacks.

When they entered the warehouse, Amir saw many more tables than in the Miami warehouse. The New York faithful—over a hundred of them—had all the guns assembled and affixed with Velcro to Yankee-logo-covered serving trays. They greeted him like royalty; everyone bowed in his presence. He spoke to the local leader of the cell, Mohammad, who showed Amir the vendor badges that each of the volunteers would wear to enter Yankee Stadium. Amir examined a logo-covered aluminum tray and was pleased with the positioning of the virus guns and their triggers on the side of the tray. The virus, Mohammad assured Amir, would not be removed from the lithium battery-powered cold storage containers, and loaded into the guns until the day of use. Mohammad reviewed the plan, going over the vendors' choreography step by step. At this point, thought Amir, it all seemed strangely simple. A thrill ran through him that it was going to happen. Tomorrow would be the big day.

Leaving the New York location, the bearded man drove Amir three-and-a-half hours north to complete the third step, this time to a warehouse just outside of Boston. Once again, Amir met with the operation's leader, approved the arrangements, and exchanged cell phone numbers. Before going to the Mandarin Oriental Hotel on Boylston Street for a much-needed rest, Amir had the driver stop at an apartment building on Van Ness Street. The building's rooftop deck would be a perfect spot from which to witness the Fenway attack. Amir smiled. In less than twenty-four hours, he would get to watch the distribution of death to 37,000 people— all from a position of safety. Shazia had vaccinated him. He was fearless. While Amir was witnessing another Boston massacre, the attacks would take place in Miami and New York at the same time. His goal: over one hundred thousand deaths on the first day.

CHAPTER 74

After an eleven-hour flight, where the three passengers got the best night's sleep they could manage, Mossad's private Gulfstream 650 jet landed at Teterboro Airport in North Jersey. Max's friend, Vinny Lloyd, the CIA case officer for the New York region, greeted Max, Ivan, and Zalman. Vinny had brought along two CIA case officers and three FBI agents. Inside a reserved room off the small Customs and Immigration reception hall, Max's team and Vinny's team introduced themselves.

"Gentlemen," said Richard Albright, the lead FBI agent, "good afternoon and welcome to the United States. Except for Dent, the two of you are guests of our government. While here, you will remain observers and sources of information for the task at hand. Max, since you're an American citizen, we cannot restrict your travel, but we expect you to stay in touch with me or Travis—" he nodded towards Travis— "until we resolve this problem. You are not functioning as an agent of the Israeli Government when you are in the United States. As you will note," and here Albright gave him a stern look, "our FBI colleagues have not yet removed you as the primary suspect in a murder case in Aspen, Colorado. There are no charges, but there is a request for you to come in for questioning. I respectfully request that you agree to an interview with the FBI once we have dealt with this current…situation."

Max responded, "We can discuss that later. Right now, we are here for one reason: we want to protect innocent Americans from dying the way people died in the attack in Tel Aviv. The U.S. Government needs our help. We will work together in teams. Once this is over," Max met Albright's gaze, "I would be happy to sit for an interview."

Taken aback by his boldness, Albright did not know how to respond. Since he didn't have a plan and needed the Israelis' information, he and his troops had no choice but to cooperate and listen.

Case Officer Lloyd asked Max, "What do you want us to do?"

Max nodded to Ivan to answer, "Well, we know that the laboratory that manufactured the viruses shipped nearly a thousand packages from an address in Germany. We could not determine the delivery addresses. We could use your help to figure out those addresses, so we can determine where the next attack might occur," said Ivan. He then blurted out, "I had access to the Federal Express IT system—" he held up a hand at Max's incredulous look— "please don't ask," and went on, "but I don't have the tracking numbers for those packages. Hopefully, you can help us get the recipient addresses."

Travis Andrews, one of the FBI agents, spoke up. "I can help you with that. If you have the origin address for the packages, I should be able to find the recipient addresses with one of our applications. Then, I'll put the addresses into another program and determine whether they are homes, apartments, stores, warehouses, or whatever."

Max said, "Thank you, Travis. That would be perfect. MacIvan, why don't you and Travis work together?" Ivan nodded, and the two of them walked out to another room.

Zalman, who had arrived with Max, spoke up after getting a nod from Max: "We will need access to a hazmat team. I suggest you bring enough equipment to outfit our entire combined teams and another two dozen agents and support people."

Then Albright said, "Aren't you getting a little ahead of yourself? You don't know for sure where the perp is, let alone whether he shipped a virus to these addresses. You're asking for a lot of expensive equipment and personnel, maybe all for naught."

Clenching his teeth tight, Max stared straight at Albright and said, "Less than two weeks ago, I saw nearly a hundred people die from a deliberate viral attack. There was nothing modern medical science could do to save them. If you want to take responsibility for an even larger number of people dying here in the U.S., that's on you. But I respectfully request hazmat suits for the three of us. MacIvan and Travis should stay here and locate likely delivery locations for the guns and viruses. We can do this without you if we need to." Max, radiating frustration, got up to walk out with Zalman, leaving Ivan to work with Travis. He didn't want to stand around doing nothing, knowing that the terrorist plan was being put into action even as they spoke.

Vinny Lloyd broke in, trying to stop the Israelis from leaving. "Max, we take this very seriously," he said, staring at Albright. The intensity in his voice rose as he continued, "especially since we do not know what we are dealing with. Now is the time that we must work as one team." Despite the resentful face made by Albright, he went on, "I'll make sure you have everything you requested immediately."

"We have a car picking us up. I hope you circulated the photograph of Amir ibn Khan to all FBI and police departments in the United States, requesting information from anybody who sees him. He is armed and dangerous and is worth more to us alive until we find and dispose of all the virus. I am sure he will be here in this country for the attack. Our goal is to find him before he kills anymore." Max let out a breath he hadn't realized he'd been holding. "Any questions?"

When no one replied, Max and Zalman left. They had no luggage. They continued walking out to the limo stop, where a black Chevy Suburban retrieved them.

Yossi, one of Max's favorite undercover Mossad agents, warmly greeted the Mossad team as they quickly piled in. Once they got on the highway, Yossi said, "Max, it was a kick driving your Porsche down to New York! We're going to pick it up in a few minutes. As requested, the weapons, ammunition, and hazmat suits are on the floor in the back seat of each car. And as you directed, I didn't experiment with any of those buttons you have on the console. That's an extraordinary car."

"It may be German-made, but it's Israeli-upgraded," Max said proudly. "RAMOW worked on it for six months."

"It looks like it can do anything."

"Almost!" Max smiled. "Thanks for bringing it down here." Then Max turned to his agents. "So, this is our plan. Once we hear from MacIvan, we plan our coverage of the likely locations. I want to be sure we have our hazmat suits readily available. We are all vulnerable."

Yossi drove inside a parking garage on the way from Teterboro Airport to Manhattan. He dropped Max and Zalman off beside the midnight blue Porsche. Next to it was a grey Lexus ES 350. Max and Zalman got in the Porsche, now bearing New York plates, and drove away. Yossi left in the grey Lexus. The Suburban, which the Israelis were sure the FBI would follow, remained inside the garage. The two cars left at different times so as not to attract attention. Max, Zalman, and Yossi met up at a Mossad safe house in Rye, New York.

As Max drove away, he recalled the last time he had seen his car, when Lilah had taken it to Hanscom Field to fly to Israel after the condo attack. It was hard to believe how much had happened since that day.

In the meantime, Ivan had stayed behind to work with Travis on the computer program. Travis signed into the FBI's desktop computer and said, "Your team leader has big balls. I've never seen anyone shoot down our Senior Regional Director. It perplexed the guy!"

Ivan chuckled. "Max knew your director was a bean counter who'd never been on the front line. So here is the list of the packages on this flash drive."

Travis inserted Ivan's flash drive into the government's desktop computer in the office of the Immigration Department at Teterboro Airport. "When this is over, you have to tell me why Dent called you MacIvan. But now, it would be great if you can find where these packages were sent. Let's see what this program can do." Travis watched as the program generated a list of addresses and zip codes from the 900 or so packages sent. From the warehouse in Germany. The next step used another FBI program to cross-reference the address list with the type of building. Ivan smiled to himself: Travis had just given the Mossad access to the entire DOJ, FBI, CIA, NCTC, and Homeland Security databases. Once they downloaded this information, one of the clever computer analysts in Israel could expunge all data related to the assassination of a terrorist in Aspen, including the photos and the reports. Max's case would just disappear.

Finding all the tracking information for the FedEx shipments took MacIvan and Travis several hours on a five-year-old Windows computer. Max had advised earlier to find locations close to the large Jewish populations. That ended up being a dead end.

"Damn it!" Travis cried out, slapping his forehead. "The packages had been delivered to addresses all up and down the Eastern seaboard of the United States. This makes it almost impossible to narrow things down to a likely attack location!"

Then Ivan sorted the data by zip codes and noticed a concentration of them in three regions: New York City, Miami, Florida, and Boston, Massachusetts. Using Travis's FBI software, he discovered that about eighty packages had been sent to three separate locations in each of the cities. A smaller number of the packages had been sent to addresses along the coast from Maine to Florida, but away from those three cities. Those destinations proved to be residences or empty buildings.

Ivan called Max and exclaimed, "You will not believe this!" He told Max what he had found.

"This is terrible," said Max under his breath. "Mac, this is what I want you to do." He gave Ivan instructions and then asked to speak to Travis.

"Travis," said Max, "you see the problem. The bastard may have planned multiple separate attacks. I want you to put those addresses on a map and see if a large public venue is nearby—a conference center, arena, something like that. My gut tells me the virus will be released in a big public space. I would propose hitting all the warehouse addresses immediately. Can you get the Miami and Boston FBI on the same page as us? I want MacIvan to stay with you to check out the warehouses there."

With Max still on the line, Travis looked more closely at the three addresses in New York. "They are all in the Bronx," said Travis. Then, suddenly, he found himself staring at his Yankees wristwatch. "Oh, my gosh!" Travis shouted into the phone. "Yankee Stadium! Tomorrow is opening day."

Max let out a groan. "Holy shit! When Mac told me the addresses of the three Boston warehouses, all near Lansdowne Street, I should have thought of Fenway Park. I've lived in Boston for nearly twenty years! The Sox opening day is also tomorrow!" Max told Travis, "I need you to get the Miami and Boston FBI Special Agents in Charge on the phone. We need to get everyone up to speed, fast."

CHAPTER 75

B y the time Travis and MacIvan had figured out the destinations of the FedEx packages, it was 9:00 p.m. The FBI teams wearing hazmat suits spread out to investigate the warehouse addresses in Miami, New York, and Boston. MacIvan stayed to work with the New York FBI. Max realized if Amir had already targeted him once, the Saudi had a personal reason to witness the attack in Boston. Zalman joined Max and headed for Boston. Yossi drove to meet up with MacIvan and the New York FBI Agents.

Driving north from New York was one of Max's favorite rides. Invigorating, cold fresh air blew in through the open windows, a product of the chilly spring evening. Old, packed snow crowded the roadside shoulders. The car could have easily held at one hundred miles per hour, but Max didn't risk it; he didn't want the police to stop him. When they stopped for gas, Zalman, in the passenger seat of the Porsche, called ahead to meet with the FBI, one block away from the first warehouse on the list. They arrived at the designated spot just after 1:00 a.m.

The FBI and the local Boston police were waiting there. Suddenly, Max recognized a tall, African-American man. It was Albert Lofton, the SAC of the Boston FBI office. Beloved by the department, he went by "Bud."

They had met eight years earlier when Max had operated on Bud's brother's heart. It took Lofton a moment to place Max.

"Hi, Doc!" he exclaimed. "I would have never guessed." The two men embraced, to the surprise of the surrounding Mossad and FBI agents.

"Sorry to surprise you like this. How's your brother doing?" asked Max.

With a big smile, Bud answered, "He's back to work and playing tennis twice a week. Since you put that new valve in his heart, he has more energy than me!"

Smiling back, Max said, "I'm happy to hear that."

Bud nodded, and then his facial expression hardened. "So, my boss instructed me to listen and collaborate on your plan. What do we have here?" he asked.

Max updated Bud and the Boston team of five FBI agents. Max acknowledged the instructions he and the Israelis had received upon their arrival in New York. "We're just observers, but we're here to help."

"Understood, Doc," Bud winked, "I hope it's ok if I call you 'Doc.' We have three warehouses to check out. I sent agents to each of the two other warehouses, with instructions not to engage but to evaluate and report back. In the next ten minutes, we should have a sense of what's happening. We'll take the lead here at this warehouse."

They left their cars one block away. The FBI agents wore earpieces for their internal communications. Max parked his car across the street, pointing away from the warehouse, which looked like a storage location for a cable company's vans and other small trucks. Bud directed two of his agents, one to the side window, the other to the front door. They spread out on foot and surrounded the warehouse.

Looking through a window, one agent saw a pile of opened Federal Express boxes strewn across the floor under the window. He communicated this to Bud. A knock on the front door by the other agent brought a man in a security guard uniform to open the door. Bud joined his agent and in Spanish asked about the boxes, which the guard duly showed him. They were stuffed with shredded paper but otherwise empty.

Afterward, Bud brought Max up to speed on what they had found. The reports from the other two Boston FBI teams seemed just as fruitless. The team at warehouse number two reported the place was empty, except for a pile of unopened Federal Express packages inside beside the front door. Warehouse three was also locked, but the team had looked in the window and saw several stacks of peanut-packed vendors' trays with the Boston Red Sox logo stickers on them. They had assumed that this was a storage space for Fenway Park.

Max glanced at his watch; it was now almost two in the morning. No wonder he was having trouble thinking things through.

Bud piped up, "The Boston addresses must be a red herring. Maybe they sent the packages here to distract us. New York was probably the only real target. I'll check in with the agents visiting the Bronx addresses."

Max closed his eyes for a moment. Suddenly, imagining the vendor trays, he thought, *What if...*

"Ask both the New York and Miami agents to see if any of the locations have similar trays with the local team logos?" Max suggested abruptly.

It took about forty minutes for the FBI teams to report back, but they found one address in each city had those logo-covered serving trays containing bags of peanuts or popcorn.

"That's it!" Max exclaimed. He was running on adrenaline now; 3:00 a.m. be damned. "They're going to use those trays to distribute the virus at Fenway!" He fixed Bud with an intense gaze. "You and the FBI agents in the other cities need to go into those warehouses."

"We would need search warrants," Bud responded.

"I can't believe it!" Max slapped his forehead. "How long should that take?"

Sensing the urgency, Bud put both hands on Max's shoulders: he didn't want anybody else to hear him. "Doc, I'm going to pull my team back," he said slowly, intimating that he would look the other way. "What

I can't see didn't happen." He let out a big breath. "OK. So, this was the Boston address where our guys saw the trays. We'll notify the other cities about what we find."

Just then, Bud received a notification from his office. The Homeland Security System had picked up facial recognition information submitted by reception at the Mandarin Oriental Hotel. They require all hotels to scan foreign passports. Bud turned to Max. "Good news. The HLS identified a face that looks like the guy we've been chasing. So they've sent agents to the hotel to check him out."

The ring on the burner phone awakened Amir from a deep sleep in the warm, comfortable bed in the dark room. He groaned and looked at the clock which read 3:10 a.m. *Did the clock stop, or did I get just four hours of sleep?* Only three people had this number. He had to answer it.

"*As-salamu alaykum,*" said Amir. He noticed a 617-area code, Boston! Suddenly, he sat up in bed.

"*Wa'alaykumu s-salam.*" said a deep voice on the other end of the line. "We had a visitor. A man drove by and stopped. He got out of his car for less than a minute and looked in one window. We didn't answer when he knocked on the door, so he drove away."

"Was it the police?"

"No, just some black car. They drove away. Maybe they had the wrong place. Only stopped for a minute!"

The wrong place at this hour? Amir was furious that they hadn't covered the windows. How stupid!

Amir screamed, "Cover all the windows now!"

Distracted by the hotel room's phone ringing, he ended the call from the warehouse and picked up the hotel extension to hear: "Good evening Mr. El-Khoury. This is the front desk calling. Sorry to disturb you at this late hour, sir, but I wanted to verify that you returned to your room tonight. I have a call to transfer to your room."

That was all Amir had to hear. Before the voice had finished, Amir had slammed the phone down and was out of bed and pulling on his pants.

He grabbed his cell phone and leather bag and rushed out of the room. A million thoughts raced through his head as he followed an exit sign to the staircase. *How did the police find me here?* he thought frantically. *I can't let anything stop my plan for tomorrow.*

The frightened attendant in the hotel's front lobby had repeated the words she was instructed to recite to the hotel guest. Before finishing the message, she watched four law enforcement officers race to the elevator and up the stairs to Amir's floor.

The Saudi ran down the back staircase from the fourth floor as quickly as possible and exited the hotel through the employee entrance on Boylston Street. He was already on the phone with his driver, telling him to pick him up around the corner on Ring Road closer to Huntington Avenue. At this hour, on this unseasonably crisp spring night, there were only a few homeless people out on the street. Shivering, without an overcoat, Amir had to wait thirty minutes before the driver arrived. At last, he jumped in the back seat, began cursing the same bearded driver for taking so long and then instructed him to drive to the warehouse.

Amir wasn't the only one in a rush. Less than a mile away, Max and Zalman got back in the Porsche and drove to the warehouse where the FBI agents had seen the vendors' trays. Max went to stand by the front door and Zalman to the window, the one through which the FBI agent had reported seeing the logo-covered trays. He reported back to Max on the comms unit that the window had been covered.

Max called Bud, five blocks away, with an update. "Listen, Bud, I want you to join us and cover our backs."

Then Max knocked on the warehouse door. No one responded. He signaled to Zalman to kick in the window as he picked the lock and forced open the front door. Max entered, crouching low as gunshots rang out. He hit the ground with his arm stretched out in front, aiming his 9 mm Beretta straight ahead.

Bud's team of FBI agents heard the shots as they pulled up in three cars. Bud sent them to surround the building. He called for police back-up as he got out of his car. On his hands and knees, he carefully crawled through the opened front door. Noticing Max in front of him on the floor, pointing his Beretta but not shooting, Bud pulled on Max's foot gently. Max quickly swung around; the Berretta cocked a few feet from Bud's face. Bud raised his hand, signaling to Max to get back and leave the building.

From his post by the window, Zalman saw Max leaving and backed away. The FBI agents had to fire three shots before the shooter inside went down. They found only two men inside: one lying on the floor, shot in the chest, the other with his hands up above his head. The Boston Police arrived with sirens blaring. Bud stood up, his weapon still raised, and saw the pile of large aluminum serving trays filled with bags of peanuts and popcorn, bathed in the glow of the police car lights from outside. He pulled his cell phone and called for an ambulance.

Amir's driver slowed to the side of the road to allow police cars with flashing lights and blaring sirens to pass. After another hundred yards, Amir looked out from the back seat and saw the warehouse two blocks away. He told the driver to pull to the side and stop in view of the warehouse's front door. Ducking down, with only his eyes and top of his head above the window-line, Amir stared in disbelief as this part of his dream evaporated. He ordered the driver to move closer to the building slowly so he could see what was happening.

Looking into the warehouse's front door, Amir saw a man emerge with a gun in his right hand. Amir recognized the doctor's face. His own face heated up with rage. *How did they discover the plan so quickly?*

As Amir's driver turned the SUV away from the scene, Amir's head bobbed up for just a moment into Max's sight line. That moment was enough. Max stared at the man who had shot Lilah, and a wave of rage roiled through him. The Masada pistol was in his hand, but the car pulled away too quickly to give him a shot at that face. Max ran for his car, calling Zalman to follow, and they loaded into the Porsche. *This time,* Max thought, *I have him on my turf.*

While they sped after Amir's car, Max called Bud on his cell. "Bud, is your team okay there?"

"Everything's under control, Doc," Bud answered.

"Good. I'd suggest calling the hazmat team to deal with the containers holding viruses. They must be there somewhere. Don't let anybody else touch anything for fear of releasing the virus."

"Thanks, Doc. I can take it from here. I'll notify the FBI teams in the other cities and let them know what we found. You and your team were right all along. Where are you going?"

Max answered only, "We're safe." Then he added, "I'll keep in touch if I find anything else. Thanks for all the help, Bud. I appreciate it."

CHAPTER 76

Max accelerated the Porsche and spoke to the digital dashboard: "Map open, local." The radio flipped over, and a large horizontal screen appeared with a local street map. After a few turns on more back streets, Amir's car appeared and headed towards Storrow Drive. Max knew that Boston's tortuous streets would make it hard to follow Amir's car from a distance. He thought of the warning that his team had received when they had landed: observe only, and do not act. *Forget about that,* Max thought. He had to see this mission through to the end.

Suddenly the Saudi's black SUV careened into view again, and Max hit a button that created a tiny target on the screen. It moved along the streets, tracking the location of the car.

"How did you do that?" asked Zalman, incredulous. "You targeted his car like a jet pilot locks in on an enemy plane!"

"Very similar technology," Max said proudly. "I've got radar with the help of overhead satellites. My car has a few tricks RAMOW created. I thought you might know about it since your friend MacIvan was the IT genius behind it."

Zalman gave an impressed nod. "Not bad, Mac!"

"Each vehicle has unique physical identifiers, or UPI's," Max explained, "which my car and the satellites track." Max smiled as he careened around a curve, squeezing the leather covered steering wheel. "Now, we can follow the guy's car without staying too close."

One hundred yards in front of them, Amir was losing patience with his cautious driver's maneuvers. On a narrow, quiet street, he ordered him to pull over. Instructed to get out, the exhausted driver willingly complied. An agitated Amir got out of the back seat behind the driver and opened the driver's door, pointing to the passenger seat. The driver got out, and Amir got into the driver's seat, locking all four doors. The tired, loyal driver trudged around to the passenger's side and tried to open the door.

The passenger-side window opened halfway. "What are you doing, sir?" the man asked. Wordlessly, feeling desperate, Amir just stared into the driver's eyes. He raised his right hand, pointing his gun at the driver's face, and pulled the trigger. Blood spurted inside the car and onto the half-closed window as the force of the gunshot pushed the dead driver back away from the vehicle. There were no witnesses. Amir put the gun on the seat next to him and wiped his sweaty hands on his pants. Quickly, he drove another block and pulled onto Storrow Drive, headed for the Southeast Expressway and Route 3 South. Distracted by the bloody mess in the car, he shook his head. *Asif would have handled that differently.*

On the screen display, the digital clock read 4:00 a.m., as Max and Zalman saw the target had stopped on a side street and then pulled forward a block to climb the entrance ramp to the highway. Max wanted to be sure Amir didn't get out. He rushed to the side street, looking for a man on the run. Instead, Zalman looked out from his passenger-side window and saw the driver's dead body on the curb between two parked cars.

"Look at this," Zalman exclaimed. Max craned his head towards the passenger side and nodded grimly. Zalman asked, "What should we do?"

He told Zalman to send an anonymous tip to the Boston Police about a dead man found in the road. Max didn't want some innocent child to discover the body on the way to school in the morning.

With Max at the wheel, Zalman's eyes followed the car on the screen. Traveling on the Southeast Expressway, the SUV drove above the speed limit, weaving in and out of his lane. Max didn't want to confront Amir on the highway. Whatever happened, he had to appear to honor the deal he had made with the FBI.

The Porsche followed Amir's car for another sixty-six miles until the SUV turned off onto Route 6, heading towards the Bourne Bridge, the entry point to Cape Cod. It appeared to Max that Amir was not just fleeing Boston: he was heading for a destination.

It was a moonlit early morning well before sunrise. Very few cars were on the road. After crossing the bridge, the black SUV speeded south on Route 28 into Pocasset. Thirty seconds behind, the Porsche got to within 200 feet of Amir. Max needed to get closer.

The Saudi pulled off the two-lane highway onto Clay Pond Road. His phone rang, and the caller confirmed the arrangement. *Shit,* he thought, *ocean again.* Amir continued slowly for another half mile to Shore Road, then pulled his car over to the side, in front of a large white cottage, displaying the number eighteen. The chilly wind blew off Buzzards Bay, forcing icy air across the abandoned beach town, whose summer residents would not return till June. There were no cars parked in the driveways and no lights on in the seasonal unheated cottages along the road.

Max stopped a block away; his lights had been off for the last two miles. As he took his hands off the wheel and his foot off the gas, Zalman was astonished to see that the Porsche continued to glide along quietly on autopilot. The gas motor was off. Moving in stealth mode, an electric motor propelled their car down Shore Road. It stopped fifty feet behind Amir's black SUV. With both cars' engines off, Zalman heard another noise. Max heard it, too. Coming from behind the cottage, maybe out in the water, it sounded like a powerboat.

"Zal, stay close to the house as you head towards the water. Be careful, he probably has a gun. I am going to see what's going on from the air," Max instructed.

Zalman understood the first part of the order. But what had Max meant by "from the air"? He got out of the car carrying his gun.

Max pushed two buttons, each with different Hebrew letters, at the bottom of the display screen. A small compartment to the right side of the rear-located engine opened, and a black drone with four horizontal propellers lifted off the back of the Porsche. In a matter of seconds, the drone's night vision video capture transmitted images to the left of the split screen on the Porsche's display.

Max watched on the screen as Amir left the car in the street and ran around the side of the house. The drone screen showed Amir heading out to the beach. A speedboat appeared and raced towards him. There may have been a shadow of another craft further out on the bay.

Zalman heard Max over his comm set: "Get down! The Saudi might see you." Zalman passed the side of the house and saw a man on the beach. He raised his gun, but not fast enough. Suddenly, a searing pain in his left shoulder knocked him to the ground. The Mossad agent struggled to find cover and kept his eye on the drone.

Shooting the man at the side of the house gave Amir a sense of safety. His hands shook from the fear of being caught. He thought about finishing the man off, but the sound of the boat and the heat of the moment distracted him. He turned to the water to signal the boat.

Max saw Zalman go down. "Shit!" he yelled to himself in the car and adjusted the drone's night vision view to display the twenty-four-foot, dark-hulled powerboat, which was now only ten meters from the beach. Max couldn't risk shooting Amir, who was too close to Zalman, so he aimed at the boat. At the push of a touch-screen button, the drone fired a small, heat-seeking rocket. Max heard it from his car and saw the sky lighting up like the Fourth of July. The boat's engine exploded, and then its gas tank blew up, burning what remained of the boat's structure. The boat's driver and another standing next to him died instantly in flames.

Remnants of the boat flew onto the sand, knocking Amir over. He lost the gun and watched his best chance for escape disappear. He hoped there was a second boat out there.

The drone hovered over Amir with a large red laser dot focused on his face and a bright spotlight illuminating him in the sand. Amir heard a man's loud voice commanding, "Stand still, do not move." Rigid with fear, Amir raised his hands and froze.

After speaking into the microphone, Max, with his nine-millimeter Masada in hand, raced around the house. After evaluating Zalman, who had been shot in the left shoulder, Max bent over and said, "Zal, can you feel your left hand?"

Opening and closing his left hand, Zalman responded, through clenched teeth, "I'm okay. I can't believe I let that guy get the drop on me."

"Get yourself back to my car. I'm going after the Saudi. You can watch from the drone's view on the screen," said Max quickly as he ran off towards the beach.

Amir was still staring up into the dark sky at the spot of red light aimed down at him. The cold breeze was blowing in from the ocean. The bright moon light cast Amir as a dark shadow.

Seeing that the Saudi was no longer holding the gun, Max slipped his pistol into his waistband and ran right at Amir, knocking him onto the sand.

Amir had not seen Max's approach and was surprised when he was knocked over. The Saudi screamed out, "You're a dead man." But found himself lying on his back in the sand with the Mossad agent over him, holding his arms down. He brought up his knees to break the man's hold and sprang to his feet.

Max wanted the Saudi on his feet so he could physically punish him in a fight. Amir raised his fists in a typical fighting stance and started to circle his opponent. "How did you find the warehouse?" Amir demanded.

Amir's elementary thrusts and kicks told Max that this would not be much of a fight. He'd let the Saudi tire himself out. "Your plan was obvious. You made it easy for us."

"But you want me alive, in case there are other such warehouses," said Amir.

"If you mean those in New York and Miami, we raided them already. No, we don't need you alive. It's okay if you die," responded Max.

The Saudi didn't like hearing that. He ran at Max, leading with a flying kick to his face. Impressed by Amir's sudden burst of fighting spirit, Max blocked the kick with his left forearm and, bending over, punched Amir in the testicles. The Saudi immediately screamed and crumpled to the ground. On the ground, clutching his crotch, Amir expected the doctor to finish him off. He managed to get up on his feet and slowly moved closer to the water.

"Are you done fighting, Amir?" asked Max.

Amir went down on one knee to appear to be struggling. He grabbed a handful of sand. Max approached the Saudi to bring him in. As Max got close, Amir stood quickly, feigned a punch with his right hand, and used his left hand to throw sand into Dent's face. Max pulled back, temporarily blinded, wiping the sand from his eyes. This allowed Amir a clean punch in the face and a sweep leg move, which sent Max crashing onto the sand.

Max had underestimated his opponent. As he started to get up from the sand, Amir attacked, kicking Max in the flank and head. Not seeing much, Max got to his feet and pushed Amir away.

Amir raced towards the water, looking for his gun. "I should have killed you in Germany like I did your girlfriend," Amir sneered at Max.

Max pulled out his Masada. Aiming it at Amir, he said, "You even failed to do that. And now it's all over. My FBI friends want you alive so they can put you on trial for attempted mass murder here in the U.S., then extradite you to Germany and Israel for murders in both countries. You are a very popular guy."

Amir raised his hands. He stared at Max. "You will never arrest me...." were the last words Max heard when he felt a crushing impact on his chest that knocked him down. Before he blacked out, Max's final thought was, *A second boat...*

CHAPTER 77

Zalman had stumbled back to the Porsche and now saw the screen displaying moving shadows on the beach. No one was under the spotlight. The low-light imaging revealed that the Saudi was at the water's edge. Max was holding a gun on him. Suddenly, Zalman heard a large caliber gun shot and watched as Max fell backward.

After seeing Dent hurled to the ground, Amir rejoiced that the other boat was close enough to take the shot. He blurted, "I am out of here now!" With Dent sprawled on the ground and not moving, Amir turned towards the water and started yelling for his rescuers to come to shore.

Zalman, meanwhile, was scrambling, fighting against the pain in his left shoulder. What if Max was dead? Because MacIvan had built the drone technology, Zalman told himself, the buttons would be intuitive. He maneuvered the drone to display the night vision scene. Max was lying immobile on his back. The Saudi had retreated towards the water, waving both hands.

The drone turned to face out in the water, and there it was: another boat with two men, one aiming a rifle. He had to do something. Zalman saw another button, a red one, and prayed that it would shoot the rocket. With the boat in the center of the drone's screen, he pressed the red button.

A target of concentric red circles filled the screen with the powerboat in the middle. In seconds the rocket found its mark, and the second boat burst into flames.

The boat blew up just as Amir had caught the rope the two boatmen had thrown to him. The explosion blasted him off his feet. He fell face-down, unconscious, into eighteen inches of cold Buzzard's Bay saltwater.

Zalman pulled himself out of the Porsche and stumbled back around the house to the beach, where he found Max gasping for breath. With one good hand, he lifted Max's head to help him catch his breath.

Max's eyes opened to see Zal. Coughing out his words, "The shot hit me," he took a deep, painful breath, "so hard in the vest," Max coughed again, "I thought I was dead."

Zalman quickly explained to Max what had transpired in the last few minutes and then helped Max to his feet. Together, they staggered to the waterline to see Amir lying face down in the water. Max waded into the water to drag Amir onto his back on the beach. He had drowned. There were no physical bruises on his head or face and no bullet holes. Ten feet out, they saw four other bodies floating.

Max hugged Zalman and thanked him. "Zal, let's take care of that shoulder," Max said. You must be in a lot of pain." Then he remarked, "My chest hurts like hell, but I'm alive. The new vest performed perfectly."

Together they made it back to the Porsche. "Max, you've got one terrific car," Zalman exclaimed. "Just tell me how to get the drone back into it."

Max chuckled, then hit two buttons, and the drone returned. "Thank God you learned to use it so quickly!" said Max. With first aid supplies in the car, Max cleansed and bandaged Zalman's shoulder wound. Using Zalman's belt, he fashioned a sling. "The wound is only in the soft tissues, but the bullet is still in you. It can wait till we get home. The bones and important structures are fine. The Porsche will take you back to Hanscom Field, where I will meet you. Best if I'm the only one here when the FBI arrives. I'll call them now."

"Fine with me. I really wanted to drive your car!" Zalman admitted. "See you there."

As Zalman was leaving, Max called Special Agent Bud Lofton and told him about Amir getting onto a boat that had exploded as he approached it. Max suspected ammunition in the speedboat might have been responsible for the explosion.

Then Max redirected his thoughts to Amir's corpse. To the medical examiner, the death would appear a drowning. Hopefully, when the FBI discovered five dead bodies in the water, they will attribute the drowning deaths to a terrible boating accident. Max was waiting alone in the front of the large white cottage on Shore Road when the FBI and Massachusetts State Police, along with the Bourne Fire Department, showed up in a blaze of lights and sirens. The explosions had gotten their attention even before Max's call.

Naturally, the drowning explanation didn't close the case for the FBI agents. When they arrived, they had a million questions for Max. He explained his soaking wet clothes by saying that he had waded out into the water to see if he could help anyone. He had been too late.

After about twenty minutes of back and forth, Bud still hadn't given up. "Let's go over this again. You chased this guy all the way here to the Cape. Why didn't you call us?" he demanded.

"I tried, but the phone access down here didn't work and kept breaking up," responded Max with a straight face.

Having trouble believing the story, Lofton's brow furrowed, and his teeth clenched. "When you got here, you found this guy running out behind the house to two boats in the water that exploded, one after the other?"

"That's about it," replied Max coyly.

"Look," said Bud, "one of the five dead guys tried to kill thousands of people in three cities. I am not disappointed with the outcome. I just want a story that will hold up when I fill out the paperwork. It has to be at least a *little* credible."

Looking straight into Bud's face, Max said, "The story is credible, I assure you. When I arrived on the scene, the guy had waded out to the boat. There were two guys in the boat. One came to the bow to assist this Amir guy. The other man in the back of the boat bent over his gas tank, apparently pumping the gas line. He lifted his gun to shoot me, and then everything exploded. Maybe the shot exploded the tank!"

"Did you shoot?" Bud demanded skeptically.

Max shook his head. I never fired a shot. Here is my gun for you to see."

Bud stared at Max, and Max returned the same flat poker face. After a full twenty seconds of silence, Bud spoke, "Well, that's the story. You'd better hope it holds up in the report."

Max then asked, "How do you plan to round up the followers who were going to carry those vendor trays?"

"We're on it, Doc," said Bud. "The man in the Boston warehouse had a list of all the names and addresses of everyone involved. He showed us devices under the trays that were to spray something, my guess, the virus. With his help, we're confident we'll be able to find all of them. Our agents in the other two cities are doing the same thing."

"That's great," Max responded, then he added, "We could use a little more help in Boston. Someone has been watching my condo building—in connection with this whole thing. I would like you to check them out as well."

"Interesting that you should bring that up," said Bud. "From an anonymous tip this morning, the FBI found five male bodies in a pile at an address in Somerville. All the victims had been suspected of terrorist activities. All were illegals. Our guys found maps, plans, and Arabic emails instructing them to watch your place and kill you when you returned. We do not know who did this—but as I said, we're not upset with the outcome."

Max felt an involuntary shudder cascade through his body. He didn't acknowledge it.

"Hey Bud, can I get a lift to Hanscom?" asked Max.

"Sure, Doc. But what happened to the Porsche, I saw you in earlier?"

"Zalman, my colleague, drove it back for me. He wanted to drive it."

Max figured that that wasn't a total lie, even though the car had driven Zal.

After getting into Bud's car, Max suddenly felt the full force of his exhaustion hit him. He dialed his favorite number and heard Lilah's concerned voice on the other end. "Hello, sweetheart," he said. "Good news! It's all over! I'm coming home to you."

CHAPTER 78

Max's cell phone buzzed, and he saw it was Dr. Simonson from Rambam Medical Center. "Good morning, Shima," said Max, "how nice to hear your voice. How are you?"

"Hi Max," said Shima, "I'm fine. The CDC and my team just finished identifying the virus that never got released in the US."

"Tell me what you found."

"It's hard to believe," Shima said, trying to calm herself as she spoke, "but the virus was identical to the 1918 virus with only one modification. The CDC had to test it in their laboratory to verify the effect of the alteration. The virus would have been uniformly fatal to anyone who contracted it. And since this virus had none of the specificity of the previous viruses they engineered, it would have infected everyone."

Max took a moment to contemplate what Dr. Simonson was saying. "Oh my God," he said. "They could have killed millions. But that was exactly what you cautioned us about in our earlier conversations. Shima, thank you for the closure on this and all your help. God, I'm so glad we stopped them."

"Max," he heard Shima take a deep breath, as if through tears, "do you realize that you and your team saved the world? Brandt and the Saudi would have unleashed an even worse pandemic than 100 years ago. Thank goodness for you and your team!"

"You are very kind," Max said. "As you know, we couldn't have done it without you. Take care, Shima. *Shalom*."

Meanwhile, in the six weeks since his arrival in Israel, Jaeger Brandt had recovered remarkably well from the brutal and mutilating assault. He had spent four weeks in a discreet military hospital getting blood transfusions, skin grafts, antibiotics, and healing nourishment. Throughout his recovery, Brandt had received the care of Israeli, German-speaking nurses and doctors. Although he never acknowledged the painstaking efforts the Israeli's made to save his life, he helped them unwittingly in more critical ways. The Israelis understood the value of stroking Brandt's ego by praising his brilliance and accomplishments. While he was on a cocktail of painkillers, Brandt's vanity, combined with his warped sense of pride, led him to disclose his secrets to the scientists from the Rambam Medical Center.

The Israeli scientists learned how he had upgraded the CRISPR technology, and the meticulous and creative procedures he had used to engineer viruses. Jaeger even divulged his most significant discovery: how he had made a virus more lethal. The Rambam researchers immediately got to work reproducing his results to treat malignant tumors in mice. Repurposing his innovations, they saw a bright future for developing patient-specific treatments for cancer.

Once Dr. Simonson agreed that they had learned all there was from Brandt, the authorities transferred him to a maximum-security private prison. The warden in charge of the lockup spent a long time discussing the doctor's fate with several colleagues, as well as the Mossad and a representative from the Prime Minister's office. They didn't want to take Brandt to trial because they didn't want the world to learn about his heinous crimes. However, he was a confessed murderer. He openly prided himself on the murders in Atlanta and St. Thomas. Brandt took responsibility for the deaths at the conference in Tel Aviv, admitting that they were all part of a greater plan to cleanse the world of undesirables. Multiple admissions of guilt made it easy to determine his fate.

A trial was unnecessary, but the Israelis still hadn't determined the sentencing. The death penalty was a legal option under Israeli law. The last execution Israel had carried out was in 1962 when Holocaust architect Adolf Eichmann was hanged for genocide and crimes against humanity. Israel's government preferred for Jaeger Brandt to just disappear. They didn't want to publicize what he had done and didn't want to offer Brandt a stage to spread his hateful ideology. The solution to this dilemma came from a very unlikely source.

The man to decide Jaeger's death sentence was a highly respected general who commanded the Sayeret Matkal, the most elite of the top fighters from the Israeli Defense Force. Israel's Prime Minister and Max had both graduated from their ranks. German-born General Wolffburg was the only non-native Israeli soldier to achieve the highest level of command. When the general heard about the prisoner, he offered to take care of the situation personally.

It was a beautiful, sunny summer day in Jerusalem for Wolffburg to go for a ride. With his driver in the front seat, the General— not in uniform today— stopped at the prison. They picked up Brandt, who sat next to the General in the back seat as the car pulled away.

Speaking in German, Dr. Brandt asked, "Who are you?"

The general answered in both men's native tongue, "I am an officer in the IDF. We met before, a long time ago."

"I don't remember meeting you," Jaeger was searching his brain but didn't recall this broad-shouldered, burly man with dark glasses set on a prominent nose.

"Let me remind you. You called me a Jew bastard as you punched me unconscious on the ground in front of our classmates at the Grundschule."

Jaeger froze, the blood drained from his face and his eyes closed tight. For a long moment, he remained speechless. His eyes opened still staring at Wolffburg.

"You have remained exactly as I remembered you," the general continued. "You were a nasty anti-Semite who had tried to kill me. As an adult, you have become a despicable character without a moral compass. Like Hitler and those who followed him, you are a sorry excuse for a human being."

"*You* have the nerve to judge *me*?" Jaeger bristled. "Look, you Jews have screwed the Palestinians for two generations! You took their land and forced them to live in poverty. Who are you to talk?"

"Don't ever equate your world with what we are trying to solve here in Israel," said the general. With that, Wolffburg swung his meaty fist across Jaeger's face, breaking his nose. Blood squirted down Brandt's face and onto his clothes. "We would never try to kill all our neighbors," he answered. "You are evil and deserve to rot in hell."

The driver pulled over to a side street, and the general grabbed Jaeger's wrists, tied them, and bound the feet together, leaving him in the back seat. Another car was there for the driver to return home. Now in the driver's seat, the general drove off onto a busy highway.

Brandt demanded, "Where are you taking me?"

"I have a special experience waiting for you," Wolffburg said, seeming to take pleasure in the words. "Death by hanging would be too easy and too quick. But I was told that you don't like dogs."

In the back seat, overcome with fear, Jaeger smelled the foul odor of his stool and urine trickle down his leg. During the weeks of skin grafting and blood transfusions, he had told the psychiatrist about his childhood nightmares. She had learned that he was deathly afraid of dogs.

They drove for another two hours until they reached the border with Syria. A pack of wild Canaan dogs lived there along the frontier, out in the open. By having pounds of raw meat left there, the General had arranged for the dogs to gather in a specific *wadi,* a remote dried riverbed. It was a natural canyon where he knew that hikers avoided the area. Also, if anyone got too close to the Syrian border, they were likely to be sniper targets.

Wolffburg got out of the car and untied Jaeger's hands and feet, noticing he still had blood crusted around his nose. Supported by the general's firm grip, Jaeger stumbled out of the car and made his way to a large, stony outcropping. Dogs barked not far from where Brandt rested on a large rock in the wadi.

Jaeger screamed, "You can't just leave me here! Those dogs will find me!"

"Yes," Wolffburg said simply, hardly repressing a smirk, and turned about to leave.

Jaeger screamed, "You Jew bastard! I wish I had killed more Jews in the Tel Aviv attack and you on the ground in the Grundschule."

Turning back to Brandt, he punched Jaeger's bloody face once again, knocking him out. If he were lucky, Wolffburg thought, Brandt would be unconscious when the dogs started on him.

"Goodbye, Jaeger Brandt," the General said calmly, standing over the scientist's unmoving body. "And for all those innocent people you murdered, may their souls rest in peace knowing that justice has been served."

The next morning, General Wolffburg dropped off his staff car for a thorough cleaning. He told the attendant that a dog had gotten sick in the back seat the previous night. The attendant laughed. The general didn't.

CHAPTER 79

MONDAY, JUNE 26, 2017
BOSTON, MASSACHUSETTS

ach ambulatory care treatment room at Max's Boston hospital contained an examination table, a desk, and three wooden chairs. This one
felt eerily familiar to Special Agent Walid Manzur. He had not been
here since he had visited his mother years ago. He didn't like hospitals. But
business was business.

Walid reached out and shook the doctor's hand. "Hello, Doctor."

"Hello," said Max. "I am Dr. Dent. How may I help you?" Sitting
across from the patient, Max stared at his face, thinking that he looked
familiar.

Agent Manzur felt his facial muscles tighten. He noticed the familiar
tension in his neck and shoulders that always arose the moment he faced
a known killer. Flashing his badge, Manzur said, "I am with the FBI. I am
here to arrest you for the murder of Asif ibn Khan."

Max stared at him. He had thought that was all over. Then he realized: *This must be the FBI agent from Denver!* "I don't know what you're
talking about," he said calmly.

"You committed first-degree murder when you killed a skier on the
slopes of Aspen Highlands. I am here to bring you to justice."

Staying seated and calm, Max realized that there was no value in denying what this man knew to be true. He confronted the accusation: "May I assume you came here from Denver?"

"Yes, I am the SAC for the Denver region," replied Manzur.

"The thing is," said Max, "you know you have no case. You don't have a body, a weapon, or a witness. And from what I have been told, there is no record in your FBI database that suggests I had anything to do with what you're describing."

"That's not my concern," said Manzur, unnerved by the doctor's reaction. *So, he isn't even going to deny it?* "I figured out your scheme, though the weapon you used is unfamiliar to me. I know you killed a man on American soil. I don't care that he was a wanted terrorist."

He wants to learn about the kill, Max was thinking. *Is he really going to arrest me? Do I need to call Bud? And then: His face is so familiar.*

The FBI agent's last name ran through his mind. *Manzur, Manzur.* Suddenly, it came back to him. *Saira Manzur,* he thought. He could picture the older woman.

Twelve years earlier, using his newly-developed surgical technique, he recalled that he had carefully carved an aneurysm out of her heart muscle, repaired the organ, and preserved the heart's electrical connections. During Saira's postoperative recovery from heart surgery, they had discussed that she and Max's mother shared nearly the same name.

"How is your mother doing?" Max asked suddenly. "Her name is Saira Manzur, is it not?"

Startled, agent Manzur asked, "How do you know my mother's name?"

"As I'm sure you remember, she had surgery twelve years ago in this hospital." Max gave a knowing smile.

Manzur could hardly shift gears in his brain fast enough to process this. "That was with Dr. Collins's team," he said slowly. Manzur thought back to the frightening time when he had almost lost his mother. He looked quizzically at the face of Dr. Dent. "Dr. Collins had mentioned a young surgeon on the team…Was that you?"

Max's smile broke into a full-on grin. "It was nice of Dr. Collins to acknowledge the team," he said modestly. "I was one of two surgeons who worked with Dr. Collins. I could never forget your mother. She was one robust woman. At age sixty-nine, she sailed through surgery like a person thirty years younger. We had to hold her back from running out of the hospital too early! I had to negotiate with her to recover in the rehabilitation hospital."

Eyes filled with tears, lips curled inward, Manzur froze in his seat.

"Now, what am I supposed to do with you?" Manzur said with a sardonic smile. "I know you are a killer. But—you are also a healer. I—" Manzur put his face in his hands and cried to himself. "I don't know what to—"

Max stood and walked over to console him. "I know how you feel about your mother. A son's love for his mother runs deep. I am sorry to have put you in this situation."

Agent Manzur looked up. "I am the one who should apologize. My superiors told me to drop the case. But I just could not let a murderer go free."

Max chuckled. "Well, you didn't. You came to arrest me for a crime no one could prove. But you solved the case, and you came all the way here. I admire you for that."

Walid answered. "I feel so stupid. Now that I know you saved my mother, I just—I think I should never have come."

Max shook his head. "Not stupid at all. First, you are a skilled detective. Second, I enjoy meeting with the families of my patients. Especially those who have had a successful outcome!"

Manzur couldn't help but laugh. He stood, about the same height as Max, but stockier, embraced Max. The two men hugged. Then Agent Manzur said, "I still can't believe you are the one who saved her!"

Max blushed. "Your mother did well because Dr. Collins built a great team. I had the privilege to work with him. He was open to new solutions for unsolved problems. Repairing a ventricular aneurysm, like the one in your mother's heart, had been fatal most of the time before we used this new technique. I am so glad she benefitted from the procedure."

Wiping his eyes, Walid said, "Thank you. Your skill to save people's lives is a gift from God."

"That's kind of you to say," said Max. "Would you join me for a coffee in the café downstairs?"

"Staring into Max's eyes, I'd be happy to have coffee with you— but first, there is something I've got to tell you."

Max waited.

"It is my fault, or the fault of my office, that you were almost killed in your apartment here in Boston. One of my now-former FBI analysts, took it upon himself to share our discovery that you were the likely killer of Asif Khan. He told someone in the Boston community and the information got back to the family in Riyadh. We have since tried to arrest him, but he must have fled the country."

Max nodded grimly. "I was wondering how they learned so quickly. Thank you for sharing that." He let out a deep breath and motioned Walid to follow him to the café. "And now, I want to hear how you figured out our not-so-clever scheme."

Walid smiled, "Well," he said as they left the exam room, "it started with the tracks left by the skis, but I do have a question about the gun you used." They talked for an hour before Walid left. Both men promised to meet again soon, in Denver, so that Max could visit Saira.

CHAPTER 80

A private jet plane left Tel Aviv with four passengers and then landed, some hours later, at Zurich's Kloten Airport. The small jet taxied to a remote area at the end of the runway and into a hangar. There, a black windowless van met the plane. The hatch opened, and an agent accompanied Domenico Bernard, with handcuffs on his wrists off the plane and into the truck.

When he looked outside, the startled Bernard asked, "You brought me home?"

Once the passenger was inside the van and shackled to his seat, the Israeli accompanying him spoke: "Domenico Bernard, you are an admitted accomplice to mass murder and guilty of acts against humanity. While we feel you are deserving of capital punishment, Israel respects the sovereignty of Switzerland, and your government requested that you return to Switzerland and be imprisoned for the rest of your natural life. There will be no option for parole."

As the van left the hangar, the Israelis returned home on their jet. As the plane lifted off the runway, one agent turned to Max and asked, "Do you think the Swiss will keep him in jail as they promised?"

Max responded, "Bernard has been a real embarrassment to his country, and especially to its banking industry. The Swiss want to keep their Holocaust complicity in the past. I wouldn't be surprised if Domenic's natural life in jail ends…unnaturally."

CHAPTER 81

Five months after Boston Red Sox opening day, Max attended a cardio-vascular conference in Vienna, with Lilah as his guest. She had fully recovered from the gunshot wound that night in Germany. The only remnant of her ordeal was her shorter haircut. She still looked as elegant as ever.

On the night after the conference ended, they dined at a fine Viennese restaurant frequented by Austria's elites. Max and Lilah had reserved a small table in the back corner for an early dinner. While chatting and sipping their after-dinner cognac, Max saw his target headed for the men's room. He got up smoothly, without attracting notice. Lilah waited for three minutes, put on her hat and dark glasses, then walked over to the table that the well-dressed Austrian man had just left.

A tall, thin, shapely woman with blonde hair to her shoulders and bright red lipstick sat alone at the table. She appeared much younger than her date. Lilah sat down across from her and, in perfect German, said, "Good evening. I know you don't know your date very well, but understand that he is not coming back, and you may be in danger if you stay." Lilah reached into her purse and took out an envelope. "Here are a thousand euros. Leave before his bodyguard returns and finds you here." The woman stared at Lilah for a few seconds, took the envelope with the money, got up, and left. Despite the chilly evening, she was wearing a thin-strapped dress, and Lilah didn't see her retrieve a coat.

Max walked into the men's room right behind Gustav and locked the door. Luckily for Max, no one else was in there. Gustav Schröder was standing at the urinal when Max came up behind him. He barely had time to turn around before receiving a hard punch just under the rib cage, which bruised his kidney. Gustav doubled over and staggered away. Stuffing Gustav's mouth with a table napkin, Max dragged him into a stall, let his pants drop to the floor, sat him down on a toilet, and pulled a syringe from his pocket. He injected a tasteless liquid down the Austrian's throat. Gustav tried to spit it out but couldn't. Looking up at Max, he choked out, "Who are you?"

Max answered, "I am Israel. You will never kill another Jew again. Say goodbye to your group of Nazis!"

Helpless, Gustav tried to hack up the liquid but couldn't stop himself from swallowing it. It was a fatal dose of potassium and digoxin; the drugs had been chosen to make it appear as a mistaken overdose of his regular medications. Max watched Gustav thrash like a pale fish. Within ninety seconds, Gustav's heart had stopped, and he collapsed on the toilet.

Effortlessly, Max put the syringe in his pocket, washed his hands in the sink, and then dried them on a cloth towel. After unlocking the door with the towel, he threw it in the bin next to the sink and walked back to the table where Lilah had already paid the bill. He nodded to her, and they strolled out, hand in hand. Their driver was waiting outside with their carry-on bags in the trunk. In a matter of seconds, they were speeding toward the airport. RAMOW knew that Gustav's bodyguard had his dinner in a cheaper restaurant at least ten minutes away. It would be a while before he returned to retrieve his boss.

Max and Lilah kept a warm silence the whole way to the terminal. Finally, after sitting down in their first-class seats on the non-stop flight from Vienna to Tel Aviv, Lilah leaned over, kissed Max, and whispered, "I hope that's the end of this group of terrorists…and it ended on 911!"

He whispered back in her ear, "Not quite. There is still one loose end: the sister."

AUTHOR'S NOTE

This book took over five years to write and was nurtured in the classrooms of Boston's GrubStreet. The story had been written two years before the global COVID-19 pandemic. The irony of the coincidence is frightening. The engineering of viruses depicted in this novel is at least a few steps ahead of present-day science. I pray that the newest technologies will evolve to cure cancers and not be weaponized.

Right-wing conspiracies are not new. But our world has taken a decided turn to the right, perhaps in response to the 60's revolution. Unfortunately, inherent in a conservative swing is a tendency towards fascism as the pendulum of politics often swings too far in one direction before it corrects. My hope is that loving values with care and respect for the vulnerable and the disenfranchised will win out.

ACKNOWLEDGMENTS

A first novel, and perhaps every novel, is never created alone. I am grateful to the many people who helped me. My editor, the brilliant and talented Dr. Michael M. Weinstein, provided me with invaluable and skillful guidance to make my writing clear, consistent, grammatically correct, and focused. Any deficits that remain in the final version are mine alone. Expert advice from intelligence agencies was provided by active and former agents and officers who volunteered to help but must remain anonymous. My friend Mehdi helped me understand the proper sequence for Muslim Prayer. Four years ago, with a draft of the story appearing on my Scrivener screen, I received critical and prescient advice from Dr. Jerome Groopman, a colleague of my dear friend Dr. Z. Myron Falchuk. Jerry suggested that for the contagion in my story, I pick a more common virus like Influenza rather than Ebola. Chairman of Pathology, Dr. Anthony Guidi, a Boston _Top Doctor_, was very supportive in sharing detailed descriptions of severe hemorrhagic pneumonia. Any clinical characterizations that stray from authentic result from the author's imagination.

I took the author's liberty of using names of friends for characters that in no way reflect the original people. Vinny, Tom, Bob, TT, AB, and others read early versions of the manuscript and provided invaluable feedback. Most importantly, I am indebted to my wife, Nancy, for her unconditional love and patience as I have embarked after retirement on a second, time-consuming, part-time career. Her expertise contributed significantly to the evolution of certain characters and chapters.